Don't shout, please !

The effect on health of noise and shouting

Ana M. Cerro

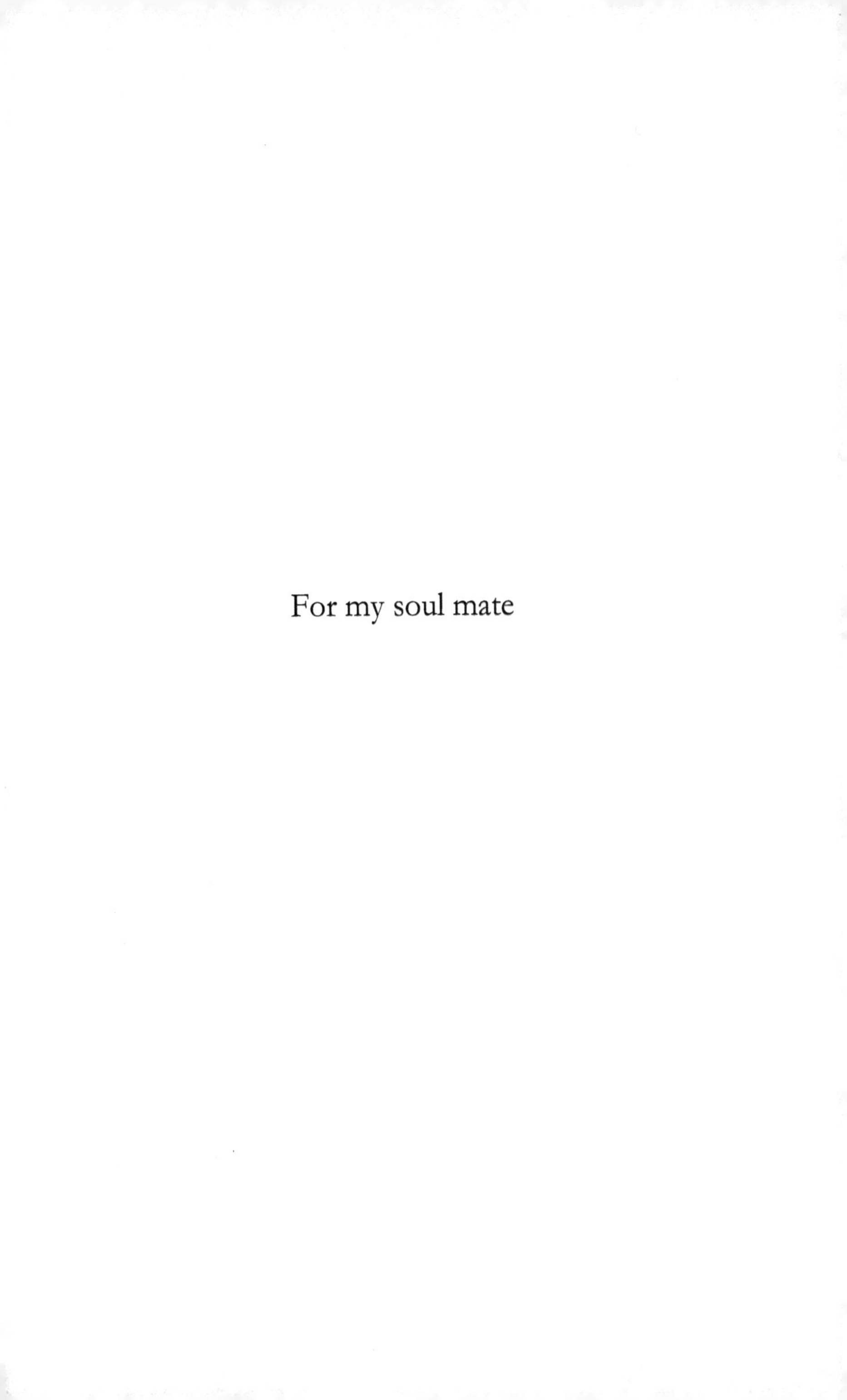

For my soul mate

Contents

FOREWORD

Health is defined as a state of complete physical, mental and social well-being, and not simply as the absence of pain or illness.[1] And this well-being depends on many factors, including noise, which is the second most important environmental cause of illness, after the ultrafine contaminating particles in the air. In Europe, for example, the majority of the people living in large urban areas are exposed to high levels of noise which are damaging to health.[2]

Noise is a type of environmental contamination which produces adverse effects on health directly and cumulatively. Moreover, the World Health Organisation (WHO) states that acoustic pollution produces adverse effects economically and socio-culturally, and also on future generations.[3]

The effect of noise on health begins with a feeling of discomfort or disturbance which manifests itself in various ways, including anger or difficulty in sleeping, which can, in turn, give rise to the production of stress hormones and to responses from the autonomic nervous system. Later, there can be disorders such as increased glucose or cholesterol in the blood, increased blood pressure, etc., disorders which can lead to certain cardiovascular diseases.[4]

But people's responses to noise can vary a lot. There are even people who live submerged in noise without regarding it as a disturbance, even though they have to make an effort to hear and respond because of it, and there are others, at the opposite extreme, who consider that noise is an intense and intolerable discomfort. I find this difference between people very curious, and it is one of the reasons which prompted my research into this subject.

I confess that I am one of those people who are sensitive to noise, and have been all my life. For many years I was obliged to study for long periods surrounded by disturbing noises produced by other people. For me it was torture hearing voices and noises invading my living space when I wanted to study or to rest. I am particularly sensitive to unnecessary noises produced by humans. When talking about noise and the environmental pollution which it produces, it is usual to consider noise from traffic, trains, factories, road works, etc., but anthropogenic noises, such as loud voices and shouts, are not included in the list of contaminating noises. However, shouting is one more noise which should be added to the others, increasing environmental pollution, and it is sometimes the main noise or the only one.

Background noises make us speak more loudly. This, which seems so obvious, was described in a scientific manner by Étienne Lombard at the beginning of the twentieth century: a person speaks more loudly when forced to do so by background noise, and when the noise stops the person again speaks at the same volume as before it began. Moreover, a person subjected to this situation does not have the feeling that they have changed or forced their voice in any way. This phenomenon, called the 'Lombard effect', is what explains why the more people there are talking in a room, the louder they talk. The loud voices make other voices louder, and the noise increases more and more in closed spaces.

As a result of the Lombard effect, the volume of one's voice increases in a room simply because there are other people's voices in the same closed space. But there are also differences which depend on the people taking part in the conversations. The din produced by one group of people in a closed room is not the same as that produced by the same number of people in another closed area, simply because the individuals involved may be more talkative or less talkative, and may speak softly, loudly or at a normal volume.

In meeting-places such as bars, restaurants, parks or terraces, and in other public places such as trains, buses, metros, hospitals, museums, etc., the level of noise can be very high — more than one might think, and much of this noise is produced by people, and their tendency to speak loudly. This does not occur to the same extent in every place and every country, so it seems that the noise and the shouts produced by individuals depend partly on them. It cannot be denied that civic education plays a large part in this, or that the way one speaks forms part of the behaviour which is learned in childhood. There is also a cultural aspect that is implicit in certain parts of the world; for example, if we consider restaurants in different regions of Europe, there are some in which people communicate almost in whispers, others in which both waiters and diners shout all the time, and others again in which the situation is intermediate.

Sometimes when people arrive in a public place which is quiet, and invade it with their shouting, the Lombard effect does not occur. Some loud voices are completely arbitrary. Some people always speak loudly. They may have hearing problems, and that may be the reason, but they themselves are not aware that they are shouting. However, we are not concerned with this here, but with people who always speak loudly without having any hearing problems (for the moment). It is possible that some people who speak very loudly or shout began to do this recently, and others have 'spoken' in this way all their lives because they learned to speak in an environment in which everyone 'spoke' like that.

It has been demonstrated that noise is a triggering factor in insomnia, stress and cardiovascular diseases, among other disorders[3]. But, as the cause of these disorders, it is usual to mention the noise produced by traffic, by industry, by transport or by road works. But what about shouting? Persistent loud voices also constitute a noise which forces us to concentrate and make great efforts to understand spoken messages and other sounds, so they are a stress factor which must first be recognised as such, especially among the 'shouting cultures', societies in which it is customary to speak loudly.

León Felipe, in the poem *¿Por qué habla tan alto el español?* ('Why does the Spaniard speak so loudly?'), from the 1940s, writes: "This raised tone of the Spaniard is an age-old defect of his race. Deep-rooted and incurable. It is a chronic illness. We Spanish have throats which are harsh and raw." This is how the poet recognised his compatriots' custom of speakly loudly. It is something that continues to be remarked on today.

I know some people with whom I find it difficult to keep up a conversation for more than ten minutes, because they speak very loudly, and I find this very tiring. They bewilder me, and all I want to do it to move away from those voices. I don't know if any of these people who speak very loudly are aware of the discomfort which they can cause. Nor do I know why they don't stop doing it, because many of them admit that they speak too loudly, yet continue to do so, and show no intention of changing the habit. Some of them even suffer from vocal problems, yet continue to force their voices; many of them end up with a disorder in the vocal cords because they have habitually spoken loudly for a long time.

It seems to me that people are not going to stop speaking loudly or shouting until they understand that, as well as being unnecessary, it is not healthy either for themselves or for others, and that shouting, like other noises, produces discomfort and stress in many people. So the purpose of this book is to review, as objectively as possible, the adverse effect of noise on health, especially of noise that can be avoided, such as shouting; of noise produced by certain behavioural habits which could be changed, thus resulting in a better quality of life for everyone.

NOISE IN THE WORLD

In the last few decades the density of the human population has increased considerably to levels unprecedented in the history of humanity, in both rich and poor countries. In 2014, 54% of the world's population was concentrated in urban areas, and it is expected that 66% will be in 2050.[5] Large urban areas are irremediably associated with acoustic contamination, so noise is going to become a problem for more people, worldwide.

Noise began to be a cause of physical and psychological stress during the Industrial Revolution. More recently, people's exposure to noise has increased even more, both in duration and in intensity, due to the ubiquitous presence of portable devices producing auditive stimulation in the form of voices, music and other sounds.[6]

I should now like to add some information which is not directly related to the main purpose of this book, but which is nevertheless interesting. It concerns a reference to noise pollution in the world which is repeated in articles in the written press and in all kinds of texts on the internet, in several languages, and which is a clear example of a large amount of 'copying and pasting' without any checking of the accuracy of the information. These texts maintain that "Spain is the noisiest country in Europe and the second most noisy country in the world, after Japan." In other versions, instead of Spain and Japan, the reference is to Madrid and Tokyo. And it is claimed that this statement is based on a report from the Organisation for Economic Co-operation and Development (OECD), produced in 1991.[7] But if we take the trouble to read that report — as Plácido Pereira Melero, a member of the Spanish Society of Acoustics points out[8] — we see a clear example of the amplification of incorrect information, because the report does not state that, it contains no information either about Madrid or about any other place in Spain, and there are only six countries for which some data (very few) are given about noise (Australia, Germany, France, Japan, The Netherlands and Switzerland). Having said this, let us now leave this fallacy aside, and continue our investigation into noise in the world. We don't know whether we shall reach the same conclusion or not, but at least we shall extract published, scientific information.

A study carried out on certain European urban agglomerations revealed that those in Germany have the lowest exposure to traffic noise, and those in Spain have the highest (the Spanish cities with more than 300,000 inhabitants, mentioned in this study, are Alicante, Bilbao, Malaga, Murcia, Pamplona and Valencia).[9]

In 2005 the first noise map of the city of Madrid was published, and the results were not very flattering: in some of the central areas the levels of noise were high by day and also at night, and in many areas they exceeded the recommended levels.[10,11]

Personal experiences and opinions in the mass media can point out the noisiest places on the planet, and they may or may not be correct. But in this review, no scientific studies have been found which compared the noise levels in different places by using the same methods of evaluation, so it is not possible to produce an objective ranking of the noisiest cities and countries. However, everyone knows where people speak very loudly and where there is a lot of noise.

Sound, noise and hearing

In physics, there is no difference between a sound and a noise. For the human ear, as the receiving organ, both are vibrations which can be perceived, but from the point of view of the person who hears them, there is an important difference. Sound is the sensory perception of the different patterns of sound waves that can be produced, for example, by a musical melody, a voice, the sound of the wind, of an explosion, an engine, etc. Noise is also a sound, but it is defined as a disturbing and unwanted sound[3], and this has a subjective element on the part of the hearer, as distinct from the purely physical phenomenon. Moreover, a particular sound can be disturbing, in other words a noise, for some people when for others it is not disturbing. But how is this possible, since the auditive organ has the same general characteristics in everyone? It seems that there is something more than physics and neurology in the perception of noise, and that the psychological characteristics of each individual play a large part.

But first, let us review some concepts of the physics of sound which will be appearing throughout the book. The parameters which define a sound are 1) intensity: how loud it is, 2) frequency: the pitch of the sound, and 3) time: how it changes with time.

The intensity or loudness of a sound is expressed in decibels (dB), defined as the level of sonic pressure, that is to say, the strength of the sound when it reaches the ear: a sound of -3 dB would be a sound of low intensity, and a sound of +3 dB would be of high intensity.

The frequency or pitch of a sound is expressed in Hertz (Hz) and determines whether the sound is high-pitched or low-pitched: a low frequency, for example, 250 Hz, corresponds to a low-pitched sound; a high frequency such as 3,500 Hz corresponds to a high-pitched sound; and a frequency of 1,000 Hz would be that of a sound of medium pitch.

But what is the human ear able to hear? It is considered that a young person with healthy hearing can hear sounds of frequencies between 20 Hz and 20,000 Hz. Sounds whose frequencies are below 20 Hz are infrasounds (between 0.02 Hz and 20 Hz), which can be heard by some animals, such as elephants, and sounds whose frequencies are above 20,000 Hz are ultrasounds (up to 20,000 kHz), which are detected by dolphins and bats and are used by these animals for echolocation (they emit ultrasounds whose sound waves rebound from the surrounding objects, allowing the animal to form an image of them).

Another important concept in the analysis of sound in closed spaces is that of reverberation, because this affects the perception of sounds and noises in those places. Sound waves, on colliding with the obstacles present in the closed space, such as walls, the ceiling, objects and people, are partly absorbed and partly reflected. After the partial absorption, the sound wave is reflected with less energy than at the beginning, but this reflected wave can collide again and continue its transmission with less energy, and so on successively. This is very important for hearing well inside buildings, and hence in the construction of meeting-rooms, classrooms, auditoria, libraries, etc. The reverberation time (RT) of a room, for a given frequency, is the number of seconds taken for the acoustic pressure to reduce by 60 dB once the emitting source has been eliminated. This time depends on the geometry of the room and of the objects in it. If the RT is short, the sounds are faint, especially if the receiver is far from the source of the sound. If the RT is prolonged, new sounds are heard at the same time as sounds emitted previously, which have not yet disappeared, and this produces distorsions and lack of intelligibility, and a tendency to increase the surrounding noise; this is what happens in some meeting-places, and it explains why the voices can become extremely loud.[12]

The other component in the transmission of sound is the receiver, our ear. The perception of a sound occurs because of the transformation of a sound wave, which is a mechanical signal, into a nerve stimulation. In the inner ear there are connections with the auditory nerve, which transmits the signal to the auditory area of the brain, which is where the signal is interpreted. But there are also indirect connections with other parts of the brain, including the limbic, neuroendocrine and autonomic nervous systems. And it is precisely by means of these connections that noise produces extra-auditory effects[12] and sensations that are different in each person.

Just as, from the age of about 40, there is a natural loss of visual acuity for close objects (known as presbyopia, or eyestrain), so also there is a natural loss of hearing with age, called presbycusis, which occurs progressively and irreversibly from the age of about 30. It is not a disease, as deafness is, but a physiological phenomenon, like the ageing of the bones or skin. In general, presbycusis is more acute when the frequencies are higher and more marked in men than in women. Hearing loss is quicker, approximately twice as quick, in men compared with women, and this holds true for most ages and frequencies.[13]

Human hearing reacts differently to the increase in sound pressure at different frequencies, attenuating or amplifying the perceived sensation: it attenuates the low frequencies (from 20 to 1,000 Hz), amplifies the high frequencies (from 1,000 to 5,000 Hz) and attenuates the very high frequencies (of more than 5,000 Hz). Because of this way of processing sound, these characteristics of human hearing are taken into account when measuring noise, and certain filters or weighting scales are applied: scale A is the one which is used the most for evaluating noise, because it is the one which most closely reflects the behaviour of human hearing. Thus, when we see information about noise, we find measurements in dB (A), which means decibels on the weighted scale A, the scale which most closely approximates to human hearing.[12]

Noise is measured with two kinds of apparatus:[12] 1) the sound-level meter, which directly measures the sound pressure and shows the reading in decibels (dB), and 2) the dosimeter, which is an exposure monitor that uses a microphone and some circuits which measure the sound pressure; the dose accumulated over time is shown on a display, and this serves to measure noises at both fixed and mobile checkpoints. These noise-measuring devices are used mainly for evaluating sound pressure at workstations and noise in different environments.

From the measurements obtained by means of sound-level meters and dosimeters, noise can be broken down into frequencies, which is important because the effects of noise, both auditory and extra-auditory, on human beings depend not only on its pressure but also on its frequency.[12]

Sensitivity to noise

A remarkable number of people use headphones while travelling by metro, bus, train, etc. Anyone listening to something by means of headphones has interrupted their auditory perception of the outside world. Some people go out wearing headphones and do not remove them until they arrive at their place of work (and some, not even then), and put them on again when they finish work. I don't know why so many people have acquired this habit, but it is something that they do deliberately, and which involves disconnecting from their surroundings. Is it because they want to listen to their favourite music or radio programme, or is it because they don't want to hear noise or voices? Perhaps the reason is a little of everything, because people have different degrees of sensitivity to noise, and they adapt as best they can to the environmental conditions in which they live.

Everyone is sensitive to noise, and this can express itself, on the one hand, as a feeling of disturbance, and on the other hand, through the effects of noise on health, such as disturbed sleep and diminished intellectual performance.

Sensitivity to noise has a genetic component[14] — it is much more similar in genetically identical (monozygotic) twins than in non-identical (dizygotic) twins — but it can also increase in certain situations, such as in people with migraine or other illnesses which affect the head, in certain mental disorders, and in infections or operations in the ears. There are also certain medicines which can increase this sensitivity.[15]

Some researchers consider that sensitivity to noise is a characteristic, an attitude, an internal state of each person which, regardless of the degree of exposure to noise, involves a greater or lesser susceptibility to it and gives rise to different reactions.[16]

It seems that sensitivity to noise is associated with sensitivity to other environmental influences such as smells, and that there could be a 'general environmental sensitivity'. If so, sensitivity to noise would be related to each person's physiology and psychology, and to a greater susceptibility to stress factors and to a negative affectivity.[17,18] But what is negative affectivity? It is the feeling of discontent, anger, dissatisfaction, etc., which some people can have. Research into the relationship between sensitivity to noise and neuroticism (the personality trait that involves vulnerability to neurosis and low tolerance of physical or psychological stress) has produced inconsistent results, some researchers finding a connection, and others not.[16] In fact, the research has not determined whether the people who are the most disturbed by noise are more 'neurotic' than those for whom it doesn't matter so much.

In connection with the relationship between sensitivity to noise and the physiological functions there are also inconsistent findings: some studies find differences in certain vital signs, such as the pulse and the blood pressure, among people with different sensitivities to noise, but in other studies no differences are found.[16]

What certainly is accepted is that sensitivity to noise is directly linked to the quality of life, at least as far as health is concerned.[19] It has been suggested that the distress caused by noise could be a factor which affects the cardiovascular system. However, the relationship between cause and effect is unknown, because the discomfort caused by noise is not the only stress factor, and there are more factors which could act simultaneously.[20]

The distress caused by noise is particularly important in connection with psychiatric disorders. And it has also been suggested that being ill can increase the degree of discomfort caused by noise, which explains why people who are not feeling well or who are ill are less tolerant to noise and to other surrounding disturbances.[20]

It has also been proposed that sensitivity to noise could be an indicator of people's vulnerability to environmental stress factors, in other words, that people who are very sensitive to noise could be more prone to falling ill when they are exposed to environmental noise.[18]

Reverting now to the habit of continuously using headphones, this could be related to sensitivity to noise, in other words, some of these individuals could be trying to alleviate the discomfort which the environmental noise produces in them by masking it with the sounds — chosen by themselves — of their audio devices. In this case, the isolation from exterior sounds enables them to actively reject the surrounding noise, while enjoying music or other sounds of their own choosing.

But the aforementioned situation very often involves risks, because these people are not aware of what is happening in their immediate vicinity. For example, cyclists wearing headphones do not notice, because they don't hear, when a car is about to overtake them; the bike moves towards the space which the overtaking vehicle is entering, and is knocked down. Nobody riding a bike or driving another vehicle should wear headphones, but some people do. There are many other moments in our daily activities in society when it is not advisable to be 'disconnected' from the sounds around us. And if noise is the reason for disconnecting from exterior sounds, then another solution must be found.

Individuals who wander everywhere wearing headphones and not hearing what surrounds them are objects which move unpredictably, obliging others to react to their capricious movements to avoid colliding with them; moreover, this type of individual sometimes does not apologise for disturbing others who, because they are not noticed, don't exist. This is selfish and anti-social behaviour which is now very widespread. So is that of people who walk down the street while speaking by mobile phone or with their gaze fixed on their smartphone, people who don't see anybody — and who disturb others — people who cross the road without looking first, focusing their auditive or visual senses on a machine, and not on their surroundings. This resembles what a robot would do. But the senses of the human body are very precious organs, which no robot could deploy in such a complex and near-perfect manner; they have enabled the human species to be alert, and thus to survive. And now, for many people, their senses are slaves of electronic devices, which they use obsessively and almost constantly. Why not stop in a fixed place, where no-one is disturbed, to speak by mobile phone or to consult it? Must everything be learned and responded to instantly? Is it not just as good, on many occasions, to hear about and respond to something a few minutes, hours or days later? How many times is it not even necessary either to receive or to answer a message?

Leaving aside, for the moment, the question of the visual and auditory alienation which is caused by these personal electronic devices, and reverting to the subject of noise, we can say that it is accepted, tolerated and even desired by some people, at least at certain times. For example, those young people who, in their leisure time, deliberately expose themselves to intense noise for fairly prolonged periods; this, which we call 'leisure noise', produces the adverse effects of noise in young people, as it does in all other humans beings, and this is logical; but this exposure brings them personal benefits, as it is a socialising kind of entertainment.[21]

'Leisure noise' is only admissible in certain places and at certain times, so that those who wish to submerge themselves in noise may do so freely, far from those who do not want this. This is something which has to be managed very well by the various local authorities, so that what is amusement for some does not become an ordeal for others.

Some people are more vulnerable than others to the adverse effect of noise on health, for example, elderly people, children and people whose socio-economic level is low.[22] Children are more vulnerable to the effects on the cognitive functions, because they are at the stage in life when learning is essential. The elderly are more susceptible to the negative effects on the cardiovascular system, and these effects can be the result of a combination of noise and air pollution. And in the poorest social groups there can be a combination of risk factors, in addition to noise pollution, that bring on illnesses, such as certain occupational activities, polluted air, the place of residence, etc.[15]

NOISE AND HEALTH

Noise can have many adverse effects, from an interference in the cognitive processes (those related to knowledge; it is explained later what they are) to a deterioration in mental and physical health.[23,24]

The WHO has pointed out that noise can be a risk to health in different ways, from auditory disorders, including pain in the ears, to unrest, alterations in social behaviour (for example, aggressivity), interferences in communication, sleep disorders and their short- and long-term consequences (such as cardiovascular effects), changes in the stress hormones with their subsequent effect on the metabolism and the immune system, or deterioration in occupational and academic performance.[25]

But in addition, a level of noise which is below that which can cause auditory disorders — a noise level which is considered as safe for the ears — can also produce changes in the body, especially when there is repeated exposure to it. For example, recreational noise affects communication and the intelligibility of what is being said, interferes in tasks which require concentration, and can cause disturbance to sleep and relaxation.[26]

Noises can be perceived differently by different people. As has already been stated, a noisy environment can irritate some people and not disturb others, whom it may even please. 'Heavy metal' music at full volume continues to delight my friend Eric, who ceased to be an adolescent quite a long time ago, but his sister Camila detests that music, saying that, for her, it's just noise, and that perhaps she feels like that because she began to listen to it at a very high volume that was imposed on her (she was referring to her brother's music at the time when they were both adolescents).

In other words, the concept of 'disturbing noise' has an obvious subjective component. As pointed out by two researchers into the psychological effect of noise, Zwicker and Fastl: "noise is not only something that can be measured with an instrument which records decibels, one must also take account of people and their ears — it is they who have to withstand the noise, whether they like it or not."[27]

It has been shown that noise has adverse effects on health and that these differ according to age. In adults, intense noise, and also the disturbed sleep caused by noise, increase the risk of disease in the cardiovascular, respiratory and musculoskeletal systems, and the risk of nervous breakdown. In elderly people, there is a greater risk of strokes, and in children, of respiratory illnesses.[3]

Noise causes sleep disturbance and disorders, and when these are chronic they affect people's well-being and quality of life.[3,22,28] Surveys of the quality of life of people living in more noisy and less noisy areas have shown that those who live in quiet areas have a better quality of life (statistically significant).[29] Living in an area which is not noisy is healthy. Moreover, if the area is a natural environment there is a better restoration of the physiological processes, perhaps promoted by positive emotions.[30]

The adverse effect of noise on health has been demonstrated by many studies. For example, it has been discovered that the greater the level of noise from road traffic or planes to which people are subjected in their homes, the greater their risk of suffering a heart attack.[31] In a study carried out in the city of Barcelona between 2004 and 2007, a relationship was found between the long-term effects of road traffic noise and mortality. More specifically, an association was observed between traffic noise and death from acute heart attack or type 2 diabetes mellitus, in men; and between traffic noise and death related to high blood pressure in women.[32]

In studies performed in Madrid, a relationship was also found between exposure to noise and death from cardiovascular disease, diabetes mellitus or respiratory diseases. It was also found that this relationship of cause and effect was closer among the elderly.[33–36] And this is of paramount importance, given that the ageing of the population in cities is progressive.

An analysis of six European countries — Belgium, Finland, France, Germany, Italy and Holland — shows that traffic noise (road, rail and air) is one of the environmental factors that has the greatest impact on health, after fine particles and the passive inhaling of tobacco smoke, which are in first and second place respectively.[37]

The effects produced by noise on humans are auditory and extra-auditory. Noise produces pain in the ears from approximately 140 decibels. The most serious auditory effect that noise can cause is the loss of auditory capacity, in other words, deafness (hypoacusis), which depends on the time of exposure and the acoustic pressure received. That deafness can be accompanied by tinnitus (ringing in the ears), which is a buzzing or whistling which people feel in their ears but which does not proceed from an external source of sound.

There is an occupational deafness, caused by noise at work, which normally results from continuous exposure to more than 85 dB.[38] But there can also be high levels of noise, causing deafness, in the sphere of leisure, as in discotheques, concerts, parties, shooting ranges, motor sports, fireworks and devices incorporating headphones, among others.

Some sports which are accompanied by loud music, such as aerobics, can permanently damage the ears, causing deafness, as can the use of headphones to listen to music, now widespread.[39,40] Moreover, deafness can result from a single exposure to a very loud noise or from repeated exposure to different degrees of loud noise over a period.[26]

Deafness caused by noise is mainly due to exposure to high frequencies (3,000-6,000 Hz). But deafness can also result from prolonged exposure to lower frequencies.[3]

The adverse extra-auditory effects of noise, which will be described below, are: 1) interferences in communication, 2) difficulty in resting and sleeping, 3) psychophysiological effects and effects on mental health and performance, 4) disturbances in the home, and 5) interference with planned activities.[3]

Noise acts negatively on the intelligibility of speech, because it interferes with the understanding of the message by masking it. In daily life, the intelligibility of speech is influenced by the volume of the voice, the pronunciation, the distance between speaker and listener, the surrounding noise and the auditory acuity and degree of attention of the listener. Moreover, in closed places reverberation also has an influence (as mentioned in 'Sound, noise and hearing'). If the reverberation lasts for more than one second, the words cannot be distinguished clearly, and the listener has to make a greater effort in order to understand.[3] And it is this failure to understand what is being discussed that causes misunderstandings and aberrant behaviour.

Among the extra-auditory effects of environmental noise, the most obvious is disturbed sleep. Uninterrupted sleep is necessary for normal physiological and mental functioning. First, noise affects one's sleep, but sleeping badly can then result in tiredness, a depressed state of mind and reduced performance the following day.[3]
Prolonged exposure to noises alters the physiological functioning of the body, and when it is habitual it produces: 1) cardiovascular effects, especially high blood pressure; 2) hormonal effects: alteration of the catecholamines (noradrenaline and adrenaline) and of the growth hormone; 3) sleeping disorders; 4) a feeling of discontent and disturbance; 5) behavioural effects: one can become irritable, have a tendency to be aggressive, with more difficult personal relationships, reduced ability to concentrate and a feeling of unease; 6) effects on communication: in noisy surroundings

the speaker has to make greater efforts, raising the voice, while the listener has to be more attentive in order to understand the message.[12]

With regard to the psychological repercussions, it seems that environmental noise does not, on its own, directly cause mental illness, but it does accelerate and intensify the development of latent mental illnesses.[3]

Later on, we shall be looking at the reality of noise in some of the places mentioned below, but first, let's consider the limits for noise that are recommended by the European authorities, which are:[26]

- Classrooms: 30-40 dB(A).

- Offices: 30-40 dB(A).

- Open-plan offices: 35-45 dB(A).

- Testing laboratories: 35-50 dB(A).

- Factories and shops: 65-70 dB(A).

- Healthcare sector: 30-45 dB(A).

Hearing disorders and disturbed sleep

The best-known consequence of exposure to loud noise is deafness, which can be due to the irreversible destruction of some of the ear's structures (both the cells of the cochlea and those of the auditory nerve).[41–43]

Loud noise can cause tinnitus[44] and a reduction in the intelligibility of speech;[45,46] moreover, it can also produce disorders in the cerebral cortex which receives messages from the ear, and these disorders cannot be detected by the test which reveals hearing disorders (the audiogram).[47] This is important, because people with disorders in the auditory cerebral cortex do not pick up sound messages even though their hearing continues to function.

Noise can make it difficult to fall asleep, can wake someone up and can also affect the depth of sleep, by a reduction of the REM (rapid eye movement) stage of sleeping, which is essential for healthy sleep. Other effects produced by noise during sleep are increased blood pressure and heartbeat, vasoconstriction and changed breathing.[3]

Uninterrupted sleep is essential for mental and physical health. The consequences, the next day, of not having slept because of noise are tiredness and a decline and poor performance in whatever activities are performed[3]. Noise has an adverse effect on attention, reading, problem-solving and memorisation (the cognitive functions). Children who live in noisy areas have increased stress hormones and higher resting blood pressure, due to greater activation of the sympathetic nervous system. Moreover, noise can produce deficiencies and errors at work, and some accidents at work are the result of deficient performance caused by noise.[3]

Mental health

Noise can produce an unpleasant feeling of anger or irritation, and can be perceived as something disturbing, a nuisance, an annoyance. After being subjected to high levels of noise for a prolonged period, a person can feel negative emotions such as anger, depression, powerlessness, exhaustion or anxiety.[2]

The WHO has stated that noise contributes to the activation of latent mental disorders. The symptoms connected with noise are: anxiety, agitation, nausea, headache, mental instability, a tendency to argue, sexual impotence, and mood changes.[3]

Noises of frequencies greater can 80 dB(A) can increase aggressive behaviour. Moreover, stronger reactions have been observed when the noise is accompanied by vibrations and contains waves of low frequency or pulses (such as shots from firearms).[3]

Sometimes, younger people, though they are not the only ones, play music on their electronic devices in the open air in public places, so that everyone present is obliged to hear their music, recordings or radio programmes. On some occasions, one of the enforced hearers will show irritation in their face, or will protest and ask the owner of the device to turn it off or use headphones. Enforced listeners do not like to hear what is imposed on them by someone else; and this has nothing to do with musical taste, but with the very fitting maxim that "one person's freedom ends where another's begins". There are many similar situations, such as that of the neighbour who puts on music, the television or the radio at full volume, disturbing the other neighbours, or that of someone who does the same thing in a hotel room, etc.

And, recalling those closed places that are shared by many people, mention must be made of those who speak by mobile telephone. Those who speak continuously, very often loudly or very loudly; some of them seem to want others to know that they are working and, yes, we realise that, because we can hear everything, but we really would prefer not to hear any of it. Some declarations, moreover, are sadder and more repulsive, as when the vociferous individual rudely confronts a sufferer who begs for the tormenting to cease. And sometimes it is not just one person who shouts through the mobile phone, but several. Exhibitionism and bad manners seem to be contagious.

Curiously, many people think that others speak very loudly when on the phone, much more loudly than they do themselves, and many people are certainly disturbed by the voices of others when they speak by telephone.[48] So the conclusion is clear: the habit of speaking by telephone in closed spaces which are shared with others should be eliminated. Go out into the corridor or the street, and find a place where you will not disturb anyone.

The WHO states that the groups which are the most vulnerable to noise, and whom the regulations concerning noise should particularly protect, are: sick people and those with disorders such as high blood pressure; people in hospitals or rehabilitation centres; foetuses, babies, children and the elderly.[3]

As has already been mentioned, it has been demonstrated that detriment to learning and health occurs in children who study in noisy environments, particularly those with noise from airports and road traffic.[49,50] But in some schools there is another kind of noise which consists of extremely loud music in the school playground. It is usually rock music that can be heard at a distance of several hundred metres. The decibels of this playground music should be measured, because they could well be above the threshold at which damage is caused to the ears. But what is the reason for playing loud music anyway? Do children need music to play in the playground and at every other moment of their daily life? Ambient music constitutes a background noise which causes children to shout even louder than many of them already shout without music.

Shouting instead of speaking, as will be shown below, causes vocal disorders and laryngeal illnesses. Furthermore, loud music can act as a stress-inducing noise, and is totally avoidable. Exposure to a continuous, loud sound can increase the feeling of defencelessness in children.[3] And background noise hinders the emission and reception of spoken messages. So playing music in school playgrounds serves no useful purpose, and can, in fact, be inducing stress in children, and difficulties in their communication and learning. It also encourages the habit of speaking loudly and shouting. In addition, loud music in school playgrounds is an imposition on hundreds of neighbours in the vicinity. This noise is avoidable, and its elimination is necessary.

Noise everywhere

The Federal Aviation Administration, the organisation responsible for civil aviation in the United States, considers that the areas which are sensitive to noise are those in which the latter interferes with the area's normal activities, and include residential areas, places where there are medical or religious activities, nature parks, wildlife refuges and historical or cultural sites, because all of those, according to this organisation, are places where tranquillity itself is part of the environment.[51] It is curious and praiseworthy that an organisation which is responsible for civil aviation should have such a considerate view of the importance of maintaining peace and quiet in those places, yet there are so many people who invade, with their shouting, hospitals and clinics, museums, libraries and places of study, cathedrals and churches popular with tourists, forests, mountains and other places inhabited by wild animals.

This lack of respect on the part of some people — too many people — for places where quietness or silence should be maintained, has become more apparent in the past few years, perhaps the past ten, fifteen or twenty years. It varies in different countries and societies, but it is something which is extending more and more, as a plague does, as the majority of human beings become more 'technological'. The use of mobile devices has become such that many of their users now use these devices everywhere, producing artificial noises and accompanying verbosity, and causing, in fact, acoustic contamination which disturbs people and other living beings in places where tranquillity should reign.

There is evidence which proves that anthropogenic noise, in its different forms, interferes in the lives of terrestrial and marine animals. Many species use forms of acoustic communication in important parts of their lives, such as the search for food or for companions of the same species. Acoustic contamination has effects on the behaviour of these animals. Moreover, noises can interfere in the reproduction, the distribution and the numbers of individuals of the different species.[52]

Some people lack consideration for the natural environment, and this is noticeable in many ways. Some, wherever they go, leave non-organic waste (glass, plastic, metal, etc.) which does not decompose by any natural process, and others, or the same individuals, inundate natural places with unnecessary sounds, whether those of their voices or shouts, or those emitted by various noise-producing devices. Why do people make noise in a forest, a mountain or another natural place? Don't they realize that they are in a place inhabited by animals and plants whose lives and ecosystems are altered by human noises? Is it so difficult to be in Nature without artificial apparatus which perturbs the environment? Sometimes these same devices, or others, are the centre of attention for such individuals who have intruded into Nature's domain, only have eyes for their machine, and only see life through it.

In short, when we find ourselves in natural surroundings we must be very careful what we do, so as not to damage them, and we must try to remain discreet, since we are merely outsiders there. In fact, we must allow ourselves to be caught by Nature while we are there, and we must not upset it.

The majority of European citizens living in urban areas are subjected to a high level of noise. The European Environment Agency states that noise pollution is a serious problem in Europe, emphasising that the main source of the noise is traffic, that noise pollution causes more than 10,000 premature deaths per year in Europe, that almost 20 million adults feel disturbed by noise, which causes sleep disorders in more than eight million of them; that every year, more than 900,000 people suffer from high blood pressure caused by noise, and that this acoustic contamination results in 43,000 admissions to hospital every year in Europe.[2]

The European Union's Environment Action Programme lists the objectives in relation to noise pollution in Europe for the coming years: the general limit for noise is 55 dB for day- evening- night, and there is a specific limit of 50 dB for the night. It is considered that, above these levels, noise produces adverse effects on health,[2] yet more than 125 million people in Europe live in environments with more than 55 dB.

People who habitually use audio players with headphones, and those who attend leisure centres, especially nocturnal ones, have a high probability of becoming deaf. Most of them are young people who in many cases don't notice anything until their hearing worsens and they realize that they can't hear very well. An early symptom of loss of hearing produced by loud music is the advent of tinnitus (buzzing or whistling in the ears). If, from the moment when the tinnitus first appears, one avoids loud noise, it is still possible to prevent the deafness from progressing.[53]

Other frequent noises are those of one's neighbourhood, coming from other homes, gardens, lifts, patios, entrances and communal areas, in other words, areas adjoining one's home. When considering the subject of noise, not much attention is paid to these sources, but they still have the same adverse effects on health as does traffic noise. And in connection with sleep, some people consider that noise produced by neighbours is just as disturbing as noise from traffic. And the most disturbing are radios, televisions, music players, audible voices — sometimes intelligible — doors banging and footsteps.[28]

The fact is that, just as with noises coming from outside the home, to alleviate the noises made by neighbours one has to spend money, on sound insulation or on moving house, and that is not always possible.[54]

The recommended good practices in relation to neighbourhood noise may seem obvious, but we should remember them and propagate them:[55]

To maintain silence and tranquillity in your life and the lives of others, apply the following measures when at home:

- *Don't disturb the neighbours with noise, either by day or by night.*

- *When using the television, radio or music player, keep the volume low.*

- *Wear slippers and never noisy shoes.*

- *Don't move furniture by dragging it across the floor, especially not at untimely hours.*

- *Don't switch on domestic appliances at night if they are noisy or transmit vibrations. Don't start up noisy toys, either.*

- *Don't carry out home improvement or DIY work during the hours of rest.*

- *Don't close doors by pointlessly banging them.*

- *Go up and down stairs without clattering.*

- *In conversations at home, avoid shouting.*

- *Inform and agree with the neighbours when holding parties.*

Here is something which encompasses all of the foregoing: "I must remember that when I make noise at home, at any time of day, I could be disturbing my neighbour, so I shall only do it if it's unavoidable. And when I know that the noise is going to be prolonged, I must warn the neighbours and inform them of how long it's going to last". This would be the ideal solution for community life.

But it seems that many people disregard the forms of co-existence relating to neighbourhood noise, and do not teach them to their children either. It is necessary to teach children that they live in society, and to tell them not to make noise at home with noisy toys, or by running, jumping, shouting, playing with balls, etc. — in short, they have to learn that noises disturb the neighbours, and to avoid producing them.

THE VOICE AND THE MANNER OF SPEAKING

People can use their voices with different intensities, in other words, they can speak loudly or softly; this is called sound pressure or voice intensity, and, as we have seen, it is measured in decibels. Another parameter of the voice is its frequency, which affects the tone of the voice and can vary a lot.

The size and shape of the vocal apparatus can affect the intensity of the voice. The mechanisms which intervene in the intensity and the tone are a combination of the action of several muscles, the flow of air and its pressure. When the subglottic pressure of the air (which is projected from the lungs to the mouth) increases, the intensity (the volume) of the voice increases.[56]

The characteristics of a person's voice are related to age, sex, profession and the society and culture to which the person belongs. And it is considered that there is a voice disorder when the quality, sonority and flexibility of a voice are different from those of the group of people of the same sex, age and culture.[57] This definition, like all definitions of normality, implies in a simplified manner that if a person's voice resembles that of people of the same sex, age and culture, it is normal.

In principle, the voices of two people of the same sex and age but from two different parts of the world could be within a universal curve of normality. But this is not necessarily so, because the frequency and intensity of someone's voice depend not only on the size of the larynx, but also on the culture to which that person belongs.[56] So the third element in the definition of a normal voice implies that a person's voice can be considered as normal within their culture but abnormal outside of it. This is what happens with the 'shouting' cultures, where speaking loudly or shouting is acceptable and is regarded as normal, but in cultures where it is not customary to shout, this is regarded as abnormal and is rejected.

The voice in different cultures

There can be great differences in oral communication between different groups of human beings. There are differences in the manner of speaking, which can be more or less direct or indirect, in the expression of emotions, in the length of time the gaze is fixed on the other's eyes while speaking (eye contact), in gestures, in the respect of turns to speak and pauses between two speakers (turn-taking and pause time), in the physical distance between them, the speed with which they speak, the amount of physical contact — touching the other while speaking — and the voice patterns. The voice pattern is determined by the volume (intensity) and the tone (frequency).

In a country such as the United States, with several cultural groups, very interesting differences have been found between the voice patterns of the different groups:[58] Afro-Americans, American Indians, Anglo/European Americans, Asian Americans and Hispanic-Americans.

Among the Afro-Americans, the intensity of the voice is very varied, from low to very high, and a high pitch is considered appropriate; communication is usually passionate and animated; the gaze is usually direct and prolonged while speaking, and less so when listening; they usually gesture quite a lot while speaking; the speaking times depend on the speaker's ability to hold attention, and the listeners usually speak when the speaker has finished; they speak at a relaxed speed, but the pause between two speakers is often brief; among groups of people there are interruptions, and one speaks before the other has finished; among friends, physical contact is frequent while speaking.

The American Indians speak with a low intensity and at a low pitch; communication is usually dispassionate, even when they are discussing something very important; looking directly into the other's eyes is considered invasive; they don't normally gesticulate; they never interrupt the speaker, and there are even silences between one person's utterance and the other's response; speaking quickly is regarded as disrespectful; interrupting the speaker is considered unacceptable and uncouth; they prefer to speak when side by side rather than face to face; and there is normally no physical contact while speaking.

The Anglo/European Americans use an intermediate pitch with very little vocal variation; communication in public is not usually emotional, in fact, members of this cultural group try to avoid emotional interactions, preferring to maintain cordiality and amiability; the speaker occasionally looks at the listener, and the listener looks attentively at the speaker; the style of speech is very direct; the use of gestures is intermediate, not as prominent as it is among Arabs or southern Italians, nor as sparing as among the English or the Japanese; speakers usually indicate that they have finished speaking by looking at listeners, but the pause is very short, and the final phrase is often merges with the first phrase of the other; in public, physical contact is minimal, and is basically restricted to a greeting handshake.

The Asian Americans use low intensity and a low pitch; expressing emotions is considered inappropriate and childish, and control of the emotions is highly valued; to express strong emotions they use indirect allusions and metaphors; the style of speech is indirect, and being direct is considered unseemly; the gaze is not fixed on the speaker for more than one or two seconds, especially when the speaker is hierarchically superior or elderly; gestures are very restricted; the length of the silences between the utterances of two people is intermediate, between that of the Anglo/European Americans and that of the American Indians; physical contact in public is almost non-existent.

Hispanic-Americans in the United States use a lower pitch and a lower voice intensity than the

Anglo/European Americans; they tend to be emotionally discreet with people whom they don't know, and they are much more expressive in environments which are exclusively Hispanic; looking directly at someone is generally considered disrespectful, especially when the person with whom they are speaking is older or has a position of authority; the style of communicating is not completely direct (this happens in the Romance languages);[59] the silences in conversations are usually short; physical contact is very frequent (as in the Latin cultures).

But it is unwise to consider that there are cultural or social stereotypes, because individuals, when alone, may have the usual behaviour of their cultural group, or they may not. But that does not change the fact that differences can indeed be observed in the general habits and customs of different cultures. So calm behaviour in public is fairly common among Swedes and Japanese, whereas Americans of the United States tend to be rather noisy.[48]

In normal circumstances, in some cultures people communicate in louder voices and speak more quickly than in others. For example, in the United States speaking loudly, with a deep voice and quickly indicates dominance and control; and in Germany the same is indicated by speaking softly, with a deep, whispering voice.[60] In China, however, people lower the pitch and volume of their voices to attract attention to the seriousness or depth of feeling in what they are saying.[61]

In Japan and China the silences in conversations are important. It is interesting to note that in the world of business, in some cultures speaking more is part of the strategy of control, whereas in others this is based on the use of silences.[60] In the Latin cultures, silences are usually regarded as a communication problem; and in situations such as sharing a lift or eating with someone without speaking, people feel uncomfortable, and prefer to exchange a few banal sentences than to remain silent.

A comparable difference is in the distance maintained between two people speaking to each other. It is greater among the Northern Europeans than among the Latins. Veronica Velo[60] gives an amusing example, involving a meeting between a Spaniard and a Dane: in the course of the conversation, the Spaniard moves physically closer and closer to the Dane, who retreats and retreats until his chair hits the wall, whereupon the Spaniard at last realizes that he has encroached into the space which the Dane needs to feel comfortable enough to converse. There are also huge cultural differences in the custom of touching (Latin cultures) or not touching (Northern Europeans), or touching very little (English, Germans, Asians).[60]

Returning now to the cultural custom of shouting — in Mediterranean countries such as Italy, Spain and Greece — the opinions and comments of many people, expressed on the internet or in the newspapers, show how irritating it can be to hear loud voices for those who are not accustomed to them. And that many foreigners living in those Mediterranean countries still cannot become accustomed to this manner of speaking, which continues to disturb them even after many years of co-habiting with it. Moreover, it seems that some of these people who speak loudly or in shouts in their own country, also do this in other countries, but many others restrain themselves, and behave in the same way as the people of the country which they are visiting.

Some people think that this habit of shouting, in certain countries, is also accompanied by bad words and swear words, and an absence of expressions of courtesy as essential as 'please', 'thank you' or asking for things kindly. With regard to this lack of polite communication, people with the same language, such as, for example, Spanish, also point out the absence of courtesy, the abuse of swear words and the high voice volume that Spaniards produce, compared with the well-mannered forms and softer tone of voice that the South Americans tend to use.

As a personal experience, I can point out that, travelling by road from France to Spain and vice versa, I have stopped many times at cafés and restaurants near the border in both countries. In the cafeterias and restaurants of France, people speak without shouting, and in those of Spain, barely a kilometre from the border, people speak much more loudly. And the most curious thing is that almost everyone speaks very loudly, not only the Spaniards, but also people speaking in other languages, who are not Spaniards, and who are probably just passing through. Why is this ? Partly it's because of the Lombard effect, no doubt, but perhaps there is something else.

Not that I have the answer, but I do have an intuition related to this. So I would like to tell the story of something that happened to me during an Easter Week in a Spanish city which, among other things, is notable for its numerous convents and churches. I was staying at a small hotel. In the morning, my companion and I were the only two people in the room for breakfast. An employee of the hotel served us breakfast and then put a radio on the floor, at full volume, with a rock song in English, and then disappeared. We waited for a few minutes to see whether he would come back so that we could ask him to turn off the radio, but as he did not come back, we turned the radio off ourselves. A minute later, another hotel employee came in and turned on the radio again at full volume and, furthermore, she recriminated us for turning off the radio. We told her that we did not want to hear it. She replied that the hotel policy was to turn on the radio while the guests have breakfast, so that they did not feel uncomfortable about talking because of the silence. We, the only ones who were there, did not feel inhibited by the absence of sounds; on the contrary, it was what we were looking for. The employee ignored us, and insisted on leaving the radio on. It was impossible to have a quiet breakfast.

This story is useful for me to point out, although this aspect will be dealt with later on, that one reason for which people speak loudly is the presence of background noises. In Spain, in cafeterias and restaurants there are usually many noises. In addition to the coffee machines and other devices and objects which can be used for the service, there is music, radio and TV with a high volume, which forces everyone to talk very loudly. This does not happen in other countries, where there is either no music or very soft music, and where, if there is a television, it is without sound.

For all the above reasons, it seems that, in some shouting cultures, where many people speak loudly, in addition, there is no choice but to speak louder because of the background noises which could be avoided, suppressed, definitively eliminated from the premises.

But within the same culture, each person will use their voice in one way or another, and not everyone will speak in the same way. With regard to health, individuals who use their voice excessively or inappropriately may suffer vocal cord injuries. The main symptom is hoarseness or dysphonia. Specifically, damage to the laryngeal mucosa (nodules and polyps are the most frequent) are related to excessive speech and voices that are too loud,[62] that is, to misuse of the voice. A relationship between having nodules on the vocal cords and having an extroverted or overactive and impulsive personality has also been observed. It has been noticed that vocal nodules are more frequent in hyperactive children.[63,64]

As has been mentioned in connection with cultural groups in the United States with a common language, the tone and volume of the voice vary between cultures. The differences between languages in tone, volume, rhythm, silences, etc., can produce totally mistaken perceptions on the part of those who do not know the language, for example, the non-native listener of a language can perceive anger or rudeness in a completely neutral or friendly conversation between two native speakers of that language.

The silences between two people conversing also vary from one culture to another. Thus, the pause time in a conversation between two North Americans is 0.74 seconds; and between two Japanese it is 5.5 seconds and can be prolonged up to 8.5 seconds,[65] something which for a Westerner could be embarrassing and produce discomfort. The opposite situation can be found in some television programmes, where silences do not exist, since the conversations overlap each other and nobody listens to anyone.

In addition, the voice also has a melody, which varies between different languages. And this gives rise to subjective perceptions of languages other than one's own. Thus, for example, an individual may perceive that other people speak in a rude or angry way in a language which they do not know, only because of the differences in phrasing, melody and intonation compared with their own language.

Another characteristic of the voice, which can differ between different countries and cultures, is time, whose musical equivalent would be the 'tempo', that is, the rhythm at which it is spoken. There are differences even between people from the same country who live in the countryside and in cities. Those who live in rural areas, in general, speak more calmly and slowly that those who live in cities.[61] Perhaps it is because the urbanites have to make themselves understood above the noises of the city and because they are always in a hurry...

Speaking and listening

The voice is produced in the larynx by the vibration of the vocal cords, which is caused by the air coming from the lungs. In addition, some parts of the body act as resonators: certain cavities of the head (the buccal cavity, the pharynx, the bony plate and the maxillary and frontal sinuses) and the thorax, which give the voice its particular timbre.[66]

The different types of human voice are classified fundamentally according to the frequency of the sound waves produced, which is measured in hertz (Hz),[67] and corresponds to the tone of the voice. The deepest voice is that of bass, with frequencies between 82 Hz and 396 Hz, and the highest-pitched is that of soprano, between 247 Hz and 1,056 Hz. Between these two extremes are, from low to high, baritone, tenor, contralto and mezzo-soprano.

But the volume or intensity of the voice is not connected with the types of voice. That is, we can speak with a low, high or normal volume, regardless of the type of voice which we have. The intensity of the voice, in decibels (dB), is controlled by the speaker, and can vary between 30 dB and 120 dB. A voice with an intensity of less than 50 dB is considered weak, the conversational voice varies between 50 dB and 65 dB, the projected voice between 65 and 90 dB — used by singers, theatre actors and lecturers, who have to project their voice (but projecting the voice is not the same as shouting) — and shouting is between 90 dB and 110 dB. Finally, lyric singers can reach 120 dB by singing, not shouting.[66]

And there is what the human ear can hear: sound with frequencies between 20 Hz and 20,000 Hz.[67] We cannot hear ultrasound (more than 20,000 Hz), like dogs and cats, which can hear ultrasounds from 20,000 Hz to 40,000 Hz, or bats and dolphins, which detect ultrasounds between 20,000 Hz and 100,000 Hz; nor do we hear the sound of the ultrasonography, between 1 and 20 megahertz (1 megahertz is 1 million Hertz). Nor can we hear infrasounds (of frequency less than 20 Hz), which elephants and moles can hear.

Continuing with the organs which are necessary for oral communication, that is to say, the larynx and the ear, we know very well when they are functioning normally and we also know what acoustic values can cause problems in communication. Thus, the ISO

9921[68] standard on spoken communication indicates the levels of quality of spoken language which are needed for an adequate understanding of messages in different scenarios, and gives the following values of conversational vocal work of the sender, measured at one metre away from the mouth of the latter: 1) a vocal work of 54 dB is a relaxed vocal effort; 2) a vocal work of 60 dB is a normal vocal effort; 3) a vocal work of 66 dB is an increased vocal effort; 4) a vocal work of 72 dB is a big vocal effort (loud voice); and 5) a vocal work of 78 dB is a very big vocal effort (very loud voice).

So in normal communication the appropriate vocal effort is between 54 dB and 65 dB. But why do certain individuals speak loudly? We can intuit some reasons, which have been confirmed by psychological and sociological studies: talking loudly can be a sign of strength, resolute behaviour, authority or social dominance, while speaking softly indicates insecurity, submission and vulnerability.[69–71] But this may not explain why there are people who talk loudly all the time, anywhere, with different people and in different situations and environments.

I worked for a time with a person who ran a department of a company and spoke vey loudly. It seemed that this person was always angry and his way of communicating seemed authoritarian. But he did not shout because of anger or to demonstrate his authority, nor because of euphoria or happiness — it was his usual way of speaking. It was quite uncomfortable for the people who worked with him, and it was embarrassing in certain situations which required restraint and discretion. This person said that he had always spoken that way and that he could not change it.

Nevertheless, unlike the person I have described, there are individuals who do ask themselves what they can do to correct this defect of speaking loudly, because they themselves recognise that it is not right. But, interestingly, there are also others who are not aware that they speak loudly and only know this because other people have told them.

Speaking loudly habitually is not a genetic characteristic, it is something acquired, which comes from a family and cultural influence. The voice of a child begins by being similar to that of the same-sex parent. The environment in which we grow up is a fundamental influence; later, depending on the subculture and the people with whom we interact, we will tend to speak in one way or another.[61]

The psychologist Guillermo Ballenato points out that we learn to speak from models. Children learn from adults how to talk to each other and tend to imitate shouts, insults or imposition if they observe these in their elders. Fortunately, children can also learn to dialogue, negotiate, and respect. Children observe and imitate actions, gestures, words, expressions, tones of voice and ways of speaking. But they don't only observe their parents and learn from them, their models for imitation are also brothers and sisters, friends, teachers or the characters of cinema and television, where one finds the largest number of individuals who speak loudly and do not listen to others. And from all these sources, the child internalises values, ideals, attitudes and forms of behaviour,[72] and all this will cause the child to become an adolescent and then an adult who will speak in a characteristic way, in some cases in shouts.

Adults change their voices to achieve better communication, but children who are learning to speak simply tend to increase the volume of voice to the level of the people around them.[73] That is why children who are surrounded by adults or schoolmates and friends who speak loudly are shouting children. The habit of shouting instead of speaking is frequent in children and it would be good for everyone to correct it at an early age, as explained in a nice way in 'The tale of speaking without shouting' (*El cuento de hablar sin gritar*),[74] recommended for children of between two and seven years of age.

Foetuses capture the sounds which surround their mothers, since the amniotic fluid is a transmitter of sound. Moreover, the foetus perceives when the mother speaks, sings, hums, shouts, cries, etc.[75] Thus, before being born, the individual is already preparing for a family life with normal or loud voices and also for sound tranquillity or the stress of noise.

Afterwards, babies also hear — except for those with ear diseases — and, in addition, they distinguish well between different voices. For example, they distinguish between voices which speak the same language as their family and voices in another language. So, what happens in the mind of a baby when it is put in environments with loud and unknown voices, together with other background noises? For example, how do babies feel in bars, noisy shopping centres, etc.? As they do not speak, or give their opinions… Does anyone think that babies enjoy these loud voices and noise? Do they look happy? Because of the increase in babies and young children in public places with a lot of noise in recent years, we might think that their parents and caregivers believe that these environments are good for them.

The reasons why people shout may be many, but in some cases there may be an exhibitionist component. For example, talking on the telephone loudly, even when the person is surrounded by strangers. This indicates two things, that the one who is speaking on the phone does not care about the privacy of their conversation and that it does not matter to them if the people who are nearby are disturbed. To prevent this lack of social respect, in some countries such as Japan, one is cautioned in trains, restaurants, bars, buses, etc., against speaking by mobile phone or using its noisy functions.

We live in noisy times. But some noises can be controlled: bells and alarms of telephones and other mobile devices, engine noise when the device or machine is not being used, background radio sound, constant music, and, also, of course, loud voices.

There are very rigorous studies which demonstrate something quite intuitive: that people shout to express very specific emotions. They speak loudly to show anger or when they feel very happy, and they speak softly in situations of sadness or intimacy. But if the situation is not one of extreme anger or happiness, and there are no background noises that oblige them — because of the Lombard effect — to raise their voices to be heard, why speak loudly?

There are some societies in which talking loudly in public is not accepted. Despite the Lombard effect, in some societies self-restraint in public places is greater, in other words, people make an effort not to talk loudly. This is something they learn when they are young: not to speak loudly in public, so as not to disturb others and to maintain discretion in front of people whom one doesn't know.

Among the publications which consider the reasons why some people talk loudly, there are articles describing situations of disputes and aggression between people, dementia and other mental illnesses. There are no studies which investigate the reason why some people speak loudly without there being a situation of anger, happiness or mental disorder. But the truth is that shouting does occur outside of these situations. It occurs, for example, in places as inappropriate as the waiting-rooms of some healthcare centres (well above the recommended noise level for the healthcare sector, 30-45 dB). In the waiting-room there are sick people, who are more sensitive to noise and who do not even want to speak or be spoken to while they are waiting for their turn. That is why, in healthcare centres, there are written and pictorial messages indicating that silence should be maintained. This is absolutely necessary.[26]

Even though there are no scientific studies which indicate a ranking of societies in which people habitually speak loudly, there are countless testimonies and opinions in newspapers and websites where people identify the cultures and nationalities whose members are "shouters", and people say they suffer from unnecessary and unjustified loud voices when they are in these countries or when they encounter these 'culturally' shouting people. And these sufferers highlight that many of these individuals, in addition, also speak a lot.

Some of the reasons why some people continually talk loudly could be: a problem in the hearing or in the modulation of the voice, a desire to oblige any strangers in their proximity to listen to what they say, to demonstrate great security (because of narcissism and exhibitionism), because the person who speaks loudly is not aware that there are others who are listening to him/her (that is, because of egocentricity), or because of a kind of inertia which leads the person to shout all day, without any relation to the different emotions or situations.

It is obvious that background noise forces us to speak more loudly, and this can have an impact on the anatomical elements of speech. There is a lot of research that demonstrates the effects of speaking louder than would be natural in an environment with less noise. An example of this is teachers, who suffer more diseases of the voice than people with other jobs.[76] And on the other side of communication, that is, in the receiver of the spoken message, the lack of understanding of the message produces situations of disadvantage and changes in behaviour; and this damage is greater in people with a hearing problem, the elderly, children who are learning the language and people who are not familiar with the language.[3]

Field studies conducted in the United States found noise levels that forced teachers to use a voice intensity of 67 dB to 78 dB at a distance of one metre from the listener. These values, as already mentioned, are considered to indicate a big vocal effort.[77] In a study carried out in Swedish nurseries, the mean voice intensity observed was 76 dB, which obliged caregivers to speak at least 9 dB above their baseline level (the level at which a person speaks with comfort, as mentioned, is less than 65 dB).[78] These are just two examples, but there are several occupations in which workers have to speak louder than normal and, as a consequence, more frequently have voice alterations, for example, singers, enliveners of groups, monitors of aerobics, shop assistants, waiters, workers in some factories, etc.[79]

The alterations in the vocal cords, in order of frequency, are: nodules, polyps, Reinke's oedema, submucosal haemorrhages, granulomas and ulcers.[80] Nodules, which are frequent in professionals who use the voice, consist of small lesions which usually sit symmetrically on the two vocal cords. They produce hoarseness and pharyngeal complaints. They are treated with speech therapy, with surgical treatment or with both.

Considering now that part of communication which is connected with the ear, we find a concept called 'listening effort', which is defined by the attention requirements necessary to understand what is being talked about.[81] According to a study carried out with two groups of adults, younger and older than 25 years of age, in which the effort that participants had to make to understand with background noise was analysed, it was observed that the effort was greater in those older than in those younger than 25.[82] This could explain why young people love entertainment places with a lot of noise and, why later, in general, this taste is lost with increasing age.

The truth is that, for many adults, listening in noisy environments is a difficult and often exhausting experience. With age, the sensory and cognitive functions, in general, are declining, but even elderly people with good hearing have more problems than younger people to understand in noisy environments.[83]

In recent years, the habit of putting background music everywhere has spread. In radio and television, for example, to listen to the news, interviews, reports, documentaries or the weather forecast, we have to concentrate on the words of the speaker, trying not to hear the background music — almost always very repetitive — that is played at the same time as the voice giving the information. Sometimes the music is loud and this effort is much greater. It can even be exhausting, and some listeners may stop paying attention. In films and television series, the background music can be constant, without interruption, to the extent that there is not single moment in which a voice without music is heard. In fact, this superimposed music masks the voices. In addition, it very often has no relation to what is being said. For example, I have seen a televised bullfighting interview, with the bulls in the background, in a beautiful estate, accompanied by fairly loud English rock music. If only one could have heard a flamenco guitar playing softly…

There is a measure known as the 'acceptable noise level' (ANL), which indicates the maximum amount of background noise that a person can tolerate while listening to someone:[84] it is the difference between the sound level of the voice and that of the background noise. The ANL varies between 0 and 25 decibels. It is considered that individuals with an ANL of less than seven dB have a high tolerance to background noise, and that those with an ANL of greater than 13 dB have a low tolerance. It seems that most people have ANL values of between 10 and 11 dB, that is, an intermediate tolerance. At the moment, no differences in ANL have been found related to age, sex, hearing sensitivity or type of background noise.[85]

In an experiment which assessed the volume of music that people preferred depending on the background noise (silence, street noise or people talking), the participants chose the highest volume of music with street noise as a background sound, the volume was lower with voices of people talking and, logically, much lower when there was no background noise.[86] This may have a reflection in real life; that is, with the millions of people who use audio devices with headphones in the street, in public transport, for sports and in other public places, and only when there is surrounding noise use a greater volume than they would in a quiet environment.

With regard to the effort which must be made to understand spoken words depending on the environmental conditions, some experiments have been done that help to better understand hearing capacity in noisy environments and certain physiological aspects related to it. Thus, for example, the way in which competing sounds can be recognised has been studied. In one experiment, participants had to recognise numbers emitted by a voice (through headphones), in situations of less to greater difficulty: listening to a number through a single ear (an easy task), simultaneously listening to a number through one ear and another number through the other ear (a task of intermediate difficulty), and series of two numbers presented simultaneously through both ears (a difficult task). The participants said the numbers which they heard and, at the same time, measurements were taken of some objective parameters of psychophysiological activity.[87] The result was that the more difficult the task was, the more the stress responses were activated, and specifically, the physiological parameters that changed the most with the difficulty of the task, that is to say, with the effort to hear the words, were the conductance of the skin[a] and the electromyographic activity[b]. This experiment serves to confirm that when one is listening, that is, hearing and understanding what is heard, the more difficult it is to understand the spoken messages, the greater the psychophysiological effort that is required.

Regarding the influence of age on hearing ability, hearing loss, especially with high frequencies (something that is more evident after approximately 60

---

[a] Skin conductance: it is the ability of the skin to conduct electricity. It is measured by placing electrodes on the skin. Emotions can produce changes in the conductance of the skin because the sweat glands are involved in it. With the activity of the sympathetic nervous system, as happens in situations of stress, the sweat glands are activated. That is why, in situations of stress, sweating occurs.

[b] Electromyography: it is a test used to record the electrical activity of muscles. It serves to know the functioning of the peripheral nervous system (the muscles and the nerves that innervate them).

years of age), produces a loss in phonetic identification and, therefore, in the recognition of words.[88,89] Nevertheless, difficulty in understanding conversations in difficult environmental conditions, that is, with noise, can already be observed in middle-aged people with normal hearing.[90–92] The effort required to understand spoken messages is greater as age increases, especially after the age of forty approximately.[92] This, in part, is related to differences in the circadian rhythm[c] between young people and older people. Young people tend to be 'evening people' and older people tend to be more 'morning people'. Young people find it more difficult to wake up in the mornings than the elderly, and the latter prefer to get up early and do most of the tasks in the morning. In general, for the same tasks — such as working or doing physical exercise — young people

---

[c] Circadian rhythm: it is the physiological rhythm that causes oscillations of physiological variables, such as hormone secretion, the sleep and wakefulness cycle, body temperature, etc., at intervals of approximately 24 hours. This rhythm is regulated by the biological clock which, in the human species, is located in the suprachiasmatic nuclei (which are in the brain).

prefer to do them and do them better in the afternoon and older people in the morning. It seems that this also happens with the ability to understand messages spoken among noises, in people without hearing problems, depending on age: the elderly understand more in the morning and young people understand more in the afternoon.[93] And this, again, could be related to the tendency of young people to congregate in noisy places in the evenings and at night, since noise is not a big problem for them when communicating.

Bars, cafes and restaurants have many sources of noise: coffee machines, television, radio, slot machines, etc. In some places they have all these devices working simultaneously. In addition, there are the voices of the clientele who, driven by the environmental noise, increase the volume of their voices; without forgetting that some people also speak loudly, and even more loudly in bars and restaurants. This is a phenomenon which exists in many parts of the world, but in view of the existing publications on this subject, it seems that there is a special interest in studying noise and shouting in bars, cafes and restaurants in some countries, such as China, the United States or Spain, where the noise in some places is extremely intense.

Exposure to loud noise is inherent in many leisure activities, especially those of young people, and can cause deafness, tinnitus and hyperacusia (reduction of tolerable noise levels for the ear). No doubt these alterations could be prevented by avoiding exposure. However, the question of whether some treatments could reduce this damage is also being investigated, with the idea of providing medicines which protect against the alterations caused by noise in the ear.

Some scientists believe that oxidative stress could be involved (as in so many other things) in the production of hearing disturbances, such as deafness, caused by loud noise. So research is also being done to discover whether some antioxidant drugs, such as a combination of N-acetylcysteine and magnesium, taken before exposure to noise, could prevent hearing damage in young adults.[94] The results of this study will also be of interest, logically, to prevent the problems of exposure to noise at work, the so-called 'occupational noise'. Perhaps using something which can prevent or reduce auditory disturbances due to noise makes more sense in people exposed for occupational reasons, since deafness by voluntary exposure to loud noise is easily avoidable, without needing to use medicines. But one can imagine that, if it were shown that some drugs can prevent the effects of noise in the ears, the companies which market them would try to get many people to consume them before going out partying.

All that needs to be investigated and discovered is a medicine which prevents the alterations of the voice caused by talking loudly. Then there would no longer be arguments which rely on vocal health to avoid the ugly habit of speaking loudly continuously.

"Bars, what pleasant places to talk..."[95] Sometimes, people stay in a cafeteria to tell each other things, to talk about their lives, but sometimes communication may not be very good. What about the messages spoken in environments with a lot of people talking loudly? To what extent are the details of the message given by one person to another in a noisy environment lost?

Studies are being carried out at the University of the Basque Country which may answer some of these questions by doing experiments which consist of a person saying a series of words in Spanish against a background of other voices (conversations of three, four, eight people), while other people, the recipients of the voices, have to recognise those words spoken within what is called 'conversational noise' (a background of people talking).[96] These experiments have detected a long list of words which are not recognised by most listeners when there are background voices. This means that in environments of people shouting, part of the communication is distorted, so misunderstandings occur. In addition, it has been proved that the intelligibility of the words is worse if the background noise is conversational than if it is of another type[97].

The noise present in places to eat and drink which are located in shopping centres, in the middle of shops and passageways, has also been researched.[98] The receiver of the spoken message in these bar-restaurants is in the middle of the noise, with a background of parallel conversations of people who are nearby (conversational noise), together with other noises coming from different sources, such as ambient music, messages from loudspeakers, the dragging of chairs and tables, objects which fall or collide, machines in operation, etc. Additionally, the quality of oral communication is determined by the intelligibility of the spoken language and by the effort of the voice.[99] In these establishments the tables are usually small and the distance between the speaker and the listener is less than one metre. Under these conditions there are studies of intelligibility in which it has been found that in some of these areas of bar-restaurants in shopping centres, the background noise is so high (greater than 70 dB) that the communication is not intelligible even if it is spoken more loudly.[98]

And now let's remember Etienne Lombard, the otolaryngologist who, at the beginning of the 20th century, described the phenomenon that bears his surname. Because Lombard was the first scientist to report that people with normal hearing speak more loudly when there is noise.[100] His studies are the starting point of all research into noise and the voice. The relationship between the sound of spoken language and ambient noise is known as the slope of Lombard, and there are many studies in this regard, from which recommendations have been drawn up — collected in the aforementioned ISO 9921[68] on spoken communication — and which indicate the levels of quality of spoken language which are needed for an adequate understanding of the messages in different scenarios: workplaces, public spaces, meeting-rooms, auditoria, etc.

From a certain number of people inside a closed place, there is an environmental noise which can exceed the levels of intelligibility. Specifically, above 70 dB of noise the quality of verbal communication is insufficient.[101]

In a study of comfort and conversational intelligibility between tables, carried out in several restaurants in Spain, it was found that the distance between the tables would have to be greater than 1.5 metres for conversations between diners at the same table to be intelligible (although the field work was done with less than 50% occupancy of the tables in most of the restaurants studied, which implies less background noise).[102] The study found that the lack of comfort and of conversational intelligibility are mainly due to constant background music or to the sound of televisions, or both simultaneously, the lack of separation between the bar and restaurant areas, the noise of manipulation of cutlery and crockery by the waiters, or the fact that the kitchens were directly connected to the restaurant. The authors point out that neither the music nor the sound of the television sets makes any sense, because people who are eating in the restaurant cannot clearly understand either one or the other and, in general, do not pay attention to them, so they are just a background noise that interferes with conversations. Eliminating these two elements from restaurants, music and the sound of television, would improve conversational intelligibility, would not involve any extra expense and is an easy solution.

Certainly, our hearing system is prepared for selective attention, and this allows us to hear what someone says while we leave aside the background sounds which do not interest us. However, this is a task which involves an effort and this is greater when the background sound is more intense.[103–105] The selective discrimination of sounds is called, in the field of research, 'the cocktail-party effect.' At first, it was used to refer to the ability of a person to understand what another person says at a party, in other words, in an environment where there are several people talking at the same time, music, clash of glasses, plates and cutlery, etc.[106] And it seems that this capacity for auditory discrimination exists in children, is highest in adolescents and is reduced in adults;[107,108] which explains why the older people are, the more they are disturbed by background noise, when they are trying to listen to something or to have a conversation. But, in any case, the ability to hear in the midst of noise has its limitations, even for the youngest of us.

Noise in particular places

Noise in classrooms is a factor which disturbs the transfer of knowledge, since, for the moment, this is based mainly on oral communication. Teachers try to compensate for background noise by raising the voice more and more, which causes them to have greater mental and emotional stress, and to suffer alterations in the vocal cords[26].

Teachers are among the professionals who have to make the most vocal effort in their work. They have to speak for long periods and use their voices to get the attention of the pupils or students. In general, they do not have time to rest from speaking because, in addition to working in the classroom, they have to continue using their voices in meetings with their colleagues, with parents, etc. In a survey of teachers in Germany, it was found that 58% of female teachers and 42% of male teachers had voice problems, and that 16% of responders had even suffered a temporary loss of voice.[26] In the United States, teachers are the professional group with the highest number of people suffering from voice pathology.[76]

The WHO guide to noise recommends that, in order to avoid communication problems, noise in the classroom should be of about 35 dB(A). Nevertheless, at present, noise levels in school classrooms can reach 60-80 dB(A), and even, sometimes, noise levels in school workshops and recreation areas may exceed the maximum recommended limits for a workplace (for example, a factory).[26]

To understand what a person is saying at a normal volume and at a distance of one metre, the background noise should not exceed 35 dB(A), and the reverberation time should be less than one second. These conditions are particularly necessary for teaching at school or for learning a foreign language.[3]

Classroom noise can be detrimental to learning, especially when the tasks include reading, or require cognitive processes such as attention or memory and problem-solving. Continuous exposure to noise in school produces deficits in sustained and visual attention in children, worse hearing discrimination, worse perception of spoken language, worse memory for tasks which require processing of large semantic content, worse reading ability and worse results in school achievement tests. And, in addition, in the studies in which children have been asked about the noise in classrooms, they have replied that it disturbs them.[109]

Most of the published studies of the effect of noise on school learning have been carried out in schools with noise from external sources (planes, trains, road traffic, construction machinery, etc.) and only in a few cases has the noise been considered as being of internal origin (air conditioning and other machinery, classrooms with inappropriate reverberation, etc.). Nevertheless, there has been almost no research into the noise produced by the pupils or students themselves. It would be interesting to know how this noise affects learning, because, in many cases, the noise produced by children in the classroom can be very loud. In a study of voice diseases among teachers in La Rioja (Spain), the majority (67%) pointed out that the noise coming from inside the classroom was, above all, that of the pupils' own voices.[110] And in a study in

Brazil, conducted by teachers who had not worked in the past two weeks due to voice problems, the majority (67%) considered that the noise existing inside the classroom was between high and unbearable.[111]

The truth is that when the classrooms are empty, the noise level is not zero decibels, which would be absolute silence. There is always a background noise, such as that of air-conditioning, which may come from the classroom itself, from other areas of the school, or from outside, as with traffic noise. Where this background noise in empty classrooms has been measured, values of between 23 and 45 dB(A) have been recorded.[109] But what happens when the classrooms are occupied by students in silence? Both in university classrooms and in primary schools, the level of noise in the classrooms with the students in silence is approximately 56 dB(A). So the mere presence of students generates noise. Finally, what level of noise is there in the classroom when students participate in teaching and learning activities? Most of the published records show levels of between 65 and 77 dB(A).[109]

The acoustic properties of the classrooms, canteens, libraries and other areas of the school are very important, since they influence the production of noise in closed places. The classroom is a closed place, so if the noise level of a classroom with acoustic treatment and occupied by students is, for example, 70 dB(A), without treatment it would be higher. The acoustic treatment of educational centres is a fundamental aspect in the context of health and noise, and for this reason the WHO has indicated some recommendations about reverberation times and maximum noise levels in different areas of schools.[3]

Noises at work are regulated by guidelines (Directive 2003/10/EC) which establish maximum limits to protect people's health. However, these guidelines were created when considering activities in which there are appliances and machinery which produce noise with many decibels, as happens in factories. But this is not the case of offices, where, in principle, the devices used do not produce these high levels of noise.

Currently, among all the annoyances which may be suffered by people working in open-plan offices, in which several people share the same space, noise is the most annoying, even though in the tertiary sector (services) the noise level does not usually exceed 65 dB(A). In this type of office the noises are multiple: telephones ringing, conversations between people, people talking on the phone, electrical devices, background music, ventilation or air-conditioning devices, noise from footsteps or from outside the office, etc.

People who have worked in individual offices and in open-plan offices say that the latter are much more uncomfortable to work in, especially for professional people whose work involves an individual effort and does not involve much interaction with other workers. The fact is that in open-plan offices, compared to individual ones, there is an increase in distraction, privacy is reduced and concentration is more difficult.[112]

Background voices in offices are common and seem to disturb many people. In a study conducted in the open-plan offices of several companies,[113] most people said that they noticed 'high' or 'very high' noise levels which were 'annoying' or 'very annoying'. But of all the types of office noise — machines, telephones ringing, intelligible conversations, unintelligible conversations and people's footsteps — the most frequent is that which comes from intelligible conversations,[113,114] which many employees hear permanently, and also consider that is the most annoying noise of all. Moreover, the second most annoying noise is that of unintelligible conversations.

But background voices in open-plan offices do not only disturb in a subjective manner, they also act on the cognitive functions of the brain. Remember that the cognitive functions include memory, calculation, language, attention, concentration, perception, recognition, orientation and the planning of activities. All of these are very important for doing one's job well. And it has been demonstrated that the background conversations in offices are detrimental to cognitive performance.[114]

The standard for acoustics in open-plan offices (ISO 3382-3:2012-2105; 2012) takes this into account and states that it is essential to reduce the noise of background voices.[115] But, are any of the conversations, which many employees notice constantly, avoidable? Are all of these conversations part of the job? Could some conversations be held in a place other than the open-plan office? Is the open-plan office the right option for people to work well?

Among the solutions for reducing the perception of background voices in open-plan offices are the following: making silent rooms available for those employees who need concentration, and other rooms for communication (cubicles for speaking by telephone, meeting-rooms, etc.), installing soundproofing systems, separation panels or walls, background music, etc.

With regard to background music in offices, it can reduce the intelligibility of the conversations,[114] which could be positive, since, as we have seen, the voices which are the most distracting are those of intelligible conversations. But what kind of music should be played? This is a tricky issue, because one type of music or melody may please some people and not others, and some types of music annoy some people and not others. And since musical tastes can be as numerous as people, background music may not serve the desired purpose of improving performance by reducing the perception of conversations. Because it has been noticed that people lose concentration whether they like music very much or whether they dislike it. So to mask conversations and, at the same time, avoid distraction, any music should be of a kind which people working in the same open-plan office neither like nor dislike.[116] It has also been found that songs, that is, music with lyrics, also distract, so they are not advisable as aids to concentration on work.[117] It's not easy, is it?

One day, in Madrid, in an Indian restaurant, I was chatting to a Swiss lady, Marianne, who was visiting as a tourist. She said that she had been stunned by the shouting in the bars and restaurants of the city, and that finding a quiet place to eat was an odyssey. She commented with relief that this restaurant was the only quiet one she had found. Finding a restaurant or cafeteria in which people do not speak loudly can be difficult in some cities and countries. For Marianne, being in public places with people shouting is torture. The stress that these noisy environments produce in her was expressed in her face, and in the way she explained her experiences in restaurants and cafes in the city. It seemed that she wanted to leave it as soon as possible and that her memories of the visit would not be very good.

The noise in some restaurants can be very loud. In some, researched in the United States, the noise level was greater than 85 dB.[118,119] But the high noise levels in these places occur in many parts of the world; it is just a matter of studying them.

In Hong Kong, the noise levels in restaurants were measured, and were between 66 dB and 82 dB, with an average of 74 dB.[120] But we should remember that with 65 dB to 70 dB of background noise there is already difficulty in distinguishing sounds, in other words, at above 70 dB of background noise, voice messages are not intelligible. Nevertheless, 74 dB of noise is a level that is below the noise limit allowed in China's regulations, which is 85 dB, which, as we have seen, is the noise level from which occupational deafness can result.[38]

The noise in restaurants may be occasional for the customers, but it is not for the people who work in them. Because, for those who serve drinks and meals is bars or restaurants, the exposure to noise is much higher over time than for the customers, because for many hours they work surrounded by noise and, in some cases, the noise level is higher than that at which there is a risk of occupational deafness.[38,118,119]

The toll of noise on health and social life

Noise, previously accepted by society as something natural and inevitable and linked to progress, has ceased to be so. The romantic idea that noisy cities are more alive is no longer very convincing. Today noise pollution in cities is a problem which affects people's health, and it seems that the main sources of this pollutant are the many kinds of transport and leisure.[38]

Noise is a factor which upsets our lives. So, in general, people prefer to live in quiet areas, to safeguard their well-being and health. And it has been proved that those who live in quiet places have a higher quality of life than those who live in noisy areas.[29] Nevertheless, not everyone has the financial means to live far from noise, so tranquillity has a value, and noise has a cost.[121]

But what about the noise of voices? The voices of neighbours, of colleagues at work, of students in classrooms, the voices of those travelling on the underground, to mention only a few. Not many people speak directly to a person who is talking loudly to ask them to speak more softly. It seems that society has accepted both the noise produced by machines and that generated by people with no self-control in their way of speaking. The media continually show sportspeople who express their joys, triumphs and failures by shouting, hitting themselves on the chest or head… these forms of expression are not justified by the release of the stress to which they are subjected, because sportspeople of other times also had their stress, but celebrated their triumphs or expressed their frustration in a controlled manner. Now, many sportspeople show a furious joy, shouting and gesticulating brutishly. And this primitive behaviour is also seen in other people. Children are learning it and imitating it: the shouts and uncontrolled gestures. This is how a shouting and hysterical society is being constructed, with individuals who only know how to express their emotions loudly.

Just as the noise of trains and planes has a social cost, so have shouting voices, although for the moment that cost has not been calculated in figures. Thus, the background conversations at work and the hubbub in classrooms result in a reduction of work and school performance, respectively. This cost would decrease if only adults at work and children at school could carry out their activity in quiet environments, without unnecessary chatter and voices in the background. This would involve a change in customs which are sometimes deeply rooted culturally, such as, in the case of adults, talking about private matters in the middle of work or, in children, continuing their games by talking and shouting in the classroom. The concentration which is needed to study and work requires one's own willpower, but also a conducive environment. In general, with some exceptions — such as the writer Vargas Llosa, who wrote some of his books amid the hubbub of certain cafés — much as one wants to focus on whatever one is doing or learning, if one is surrounded by people talking, concentration is more difficult and sometimes impossible, as well as frustrating.

In 2003, García Sanz and Garrido pointed out that "Living in societies which produce more and more noise is going to be increasingly expensive, because noise can only be alleviated or mitigated by heavy investments for which states and citizens have to be prepared."[38] And this is a reality — there are people who have to move house because of noise, or who have to instal acoustic insulation in their homes, etc.

The European Environment Agency includes, in its latest report about noise in Europe, an estimate of the social cost resulting from the noise of rail and road traffic in the European Union at €40 million per year, 90% of which is attributed to cars and goods vehicles.[2]

But it would be very interesting to know what the socio-health cost of the shouting voices is. This cost would include the expenses resulting from the pathology of the voice and the ear related to the use and reception of loud voices, respectively. The healthcare cost of the vocal pathology would include the cost of the visits of the person with dysphonia for general medicine, of the visits to the specialist, of diagnostic tests, of treatments and of speech therapy. In addition, we should add the healthcare costs caused by sleep disturbances and those caused by stress. These expenses would be more difficult to calculate because, in general, several factors tend to intervene in the development of these disorders, in addition to loud voices and noise. Besides, the social cost would have to include absences from work and school due to the alterations of the voice and the ear caused by noise and, especially, by shouting voices, as well as the losses of productivity and performance at work and in study centres due to background voices.

There are some studies related to the economic burden of dysphonia, one of the main symptoms of laryngeal pathology caused by the misuse of the voice. On the one hand, it has been reported that 7.2% of absence from work for one or more days per year in the general population is due to voice problems.[122] In addition, it has been shown that dysphonia has negative effects on the quality of life due to the deterioration of communication, social isolation and depression; and that it produces a negative impact on productivity at work.[123] In 2012, it was calculated that the direct costs of dysphonia (healthcare and surgical and pharmacological treatments) were between €500 and €820 per person per year.[124]

Deafness caused by exposure to noise is a health problem which has not been quantified in financial terms. But it is obvious that hearing loss in children can have a great negative effect on the learning and communication processes. There are some studies, in adults, of the costs due to the loss of quality of life and of production in workers with deafness caused by noise.[125] In any case, the costs related to hearing loss resulting from noise should also include both the healthcare costs and those related to the psychosocial effects of hearing loss.

And finally, pleasant voices

I have not found any scientific studies which have researched into why some people, families or societies speak loudly or very loudly in all circumstances. But I think that research could be carried out into the reasons why some individuals — without hearing problems or speech or psychiatric disorders — habitually talk to each other loudly outside a situation of happiness or anger. It would be interesting to know how many people do this because they don't care about other people, how many due to exhibitionism, and how many for both reasons, and whether there are people who do not do this for any of these reasons, but do know why they speak loudly. It would also be important to know if they have any idea of the negative effects on health that can be caused by shouting, both for those who speak loudly all the time, and for those who have no choice but to hear them.

In normal situations, without any drama, people who speak with temperance, without fuss or loud voices, are understood well, and others pay attention to them. Listening to some voices is a pleasure. The taste for one voice or another depends on each person, but listening, on radio or television, to a voice with good intonation and which articulates the words is ideal for everyone. This is especially important in the news. Moreover, voice messages are better understood without background sounds, such as music. The latter should be used in a measured way, selecting the type and volume very well, always taking into account that the listeners basically want to hear the spoken message, so the music should not interfere with this.

Although there are no specific studies of the harmful effect of shouting on health, it can be inferred that from a certain level of noise it is harmful, just as a high decibel level produced by machines in factories, planes, cars, etc., is harmful to health. And the fact that noise reaches levels which are harmful to health affects many people, such as those who work in bars, cafés and restaurants, users of waiting-rooms in different places or users of shared work areas.

In everyday life, a speaker does not have to project the words as in a theatrical performance, so that everyone can hear him/her, even those in the back row. One just has to talk so that the person or people with whom one is communicating can understand, not so as to be heard at several metres' distance. The loud voices which are used in some television programmes, assemblies, demonstrations, etc., are not necessary at most moments of daily life, and are, on the contrary, an inconvenience in many activities, situations and places. Speaking loudly should be avoided in certain places such as healthcare centres, shared areas such as public transport, libraries, museums, hotels and non-detached homes, since it causes great discomfort and stress in many people, and affects their health. And loud voices and shouting in natural areas should also disappear, as a measure of respect for the living beings which inhabit them, and for their protection.

I have not found any studies which explain why there are people who speak loudly or shout all the time, and why this happens especially in some cultures, but I think it would be good to research it with fieldwork, from psychological and sociological approaches, but also from a perspective of healthcare and social cost. Moreover, it is something about which almost everyone has some idea or opinion, so my next step, in my modest research about speaking loudly, will be to see how people who want to can contribute ideas and opinions.

REFERENCES

1. Preamble to the Constitution of the World Health Organization as adopted by the International Health Conference, New York, 19-22 June, 1946; signed on 22 July 1946 by the representatives of 61 States (Official Records of the World Health Organization, no. 2, p. 100) and entered into force on 7 April 1948.

2. European Environment Agency. Noise in Europe 2014 [Internet]. Luxembourg: Publications Office; 2014 [cited 2015 Jul 28]. Available from: http://bookshop.europa.eu/uri?target=EUB:NOTICE:THAL14010:EN:HTML

3. Berglund B, Lindvall T, Schwela DH. Guidelines for community noise. World Health Organization, Geneva [Internet]. 1999 [cited 2015 May 6]. Available from: http://whqlibdoc.who.int/hq/1999/a68672.pdf?ua=1

4. European Environment Agency. Good practice guide on noise exposure and potential health effects. [Internet]. Luxembourg: Publications Office; 2010 [cited 2015 May 6]. Available from: http://dx.publications.europa.eu/10.2800/54080

5. UN: World Urbanization Prospects: The 2014 Revision. United Nations, New York; 2015.

6. Szalma JL, Hancock PA. Noise effects on human performance: A meta-analytic synthesis. Psychol Bull. 2011;137(4):682–707.

7. OCDE. Lutter contre le bruit dans les années 90. Paris: OECD; 1991. 319 p.

8. Pereira Melero P. Falsa leyenda: Madrid es la ciudad más ruidosa después... Rev Esp Acústica. 2011;42(1 y 2):68–70.

9. Arana M, San Martin R, Salinas JC. People exposed to traffic noise in European agglomerations from noise maps. A

critical review. Noise Mapp [Internet]. 2014 [cited 2015 May 8];1(1). Available from: http://www.degruyter.com/view/j/noise.2014.1.issue-1/noise-2014-0005/noise-2014-0005.xml

10.   Moreno Jiménez A, Martínez Suárez P. El ruido ambiental urbano en Madrid. Caracterización y evaluación cuantitativa de la población potencialmente afectable. Bol Asoc Geógrafos Esp. 2005;40:153–79.

11.   Martínez P, Moreno A. Análisis espacio-temporal con SIG del ruido ambiental urbano en Madrid y sus distritos. Rev Int Cienc Tecnol Inf Geográfica. 2005;(5):219–249.

12.   Álvarez Bayona T. Aspectos Ergonómicos del Ruido [Internet]. Centro Nacional de Nuevas Tecnologías. Instituto Nacional de Seguridad Social e Higiene en el Trabajo; [cited 2015 May 13]. Available from: http://www.insht.es/Ergonomia2/Contenidos/Promocion ales/Ruido%20y%20Vibraciones/ficheros/DTE-AspectosErgonomicosRUIDOVIBRACIONES.pdf

13.   Pearson JD, Morrell CH, Gordon-Salant S, Brant LJ, Metter EJ, Klein LL, et al. Gender differences in a longitudinal study of age-associated hearing loss. J Acoust Soc Am. 1995;97(2):1196–205.

14.   Heinonen-Guzejev M, Vuorinen HS, Mussalo-Rauhamaa H, Heikkilä K, Koskenvuo M, Kaprio J. Genetic component of noise sensitivity. Twin Res Hum Genet Off J Int Soc Twin Stud. 2005 Jun;8(3):245–9.

15.   van Kamp I, Davies H. Noise and health in vulnerable groups: A review. Noise Health. 2013;15(64):153–9.

16.   Schreckenberg D, Griefahn B, Meis M. The associations between noise sensitivity, reported physical and mental health, perceived environmental quality, and noise annoyance. Noise Health. 2010;12(46):7–16.

17.   Stansfeld SA, Sharp DS, Gallacher J, Babisch W. Road traffic noise, noise sensitivity and psychological disorder. Psychol Med. 1993;23(4):977–85.

18. Stansfeld SA. Noise, noise sensitivity and psychiatric disorder: epidemiological and psychophysiological studies. Psychol Med. 1992;Suppl 22:1–44.

19. Shepherd D, Welch D, Dirks KN, Mathews R. Exploring the Relationship between Noise Sensitivity, Annoyance and Health-Related Quality of Life in a Sample of Adults Exposed to Environmental Noise. Int J Environ Res Public Health. 2010;7(10):3579–94.

20. Stansfeld SA, Shipley M. Noise sensitivity and future risk of illness and mortality. Sci Total Environ. 2015;520:114–9.

21. Martimportugués Goyenechea C, Luque Pons VM. Estilos de ocio y ruido. Rev Acústica. 2014;45(1–2):25–34.

22. Theakston F, editor. Burden of disease from environmental noise: quantification of healthy life years lost in Europe. Copenhagen: World Health Organization, Regional Office for Europe; 2011. 106 p.

23. Smith AP. The effects of noise and time on task on recall of order information. Br J Psychol. 1983;74:83–9.

24. Clark, C. R. (1984). The effects of noise on health. In D. M. Jones & A. J. Chapman (Eds.), Noise and society (pp. 111–124). New York, NY: Wiley [Internet]. [cited 2016 Jul 6]. Available from: http://kungfu.psy.cmu.edu/~scohen/noisechap84.pdf

25. Data and statistics. Noise and health resources. WHO website [Internet]. 2016 [cited 2016 Jul 4]. Available from: http://www.euro.who.int/en/health-topics/environment-and-health/noise/data-and-statistics

26. Schneider E, Paoli P, Brun E, European Agency for Safety and Health at Work, editors. Noise in figures. Luxembourg: Office for Official Publications of the European Communities; 2005. 116 p.

27. Zwicker E, Fastl H. Psychoacoustics: facts and models, 3rd ed.: Springer: Heidelberg, Germany,1999 [Internet]. [cited 2016 Apr 15]. Available from: http://trove.nla.gov.au/work/6331315

28.   Hurtley C, World Health Organization, editors. Night noise guidelines for Europe. Copenhagen, Denmark: World Health Organization Europe; 2009. 162 p.

29.   Shepherd D, Welch D, Dirks K, McBride D. Do Quiet Areas Afford Greater Health-Related Quality of Life than Noisy Areas? Int J Env Res Public Health. 2013;10:1284–303.

30.   Ulrich RS, Simons RF, Losito BD, Fiorito E, Miles MA, Zelson M. Stress Recovery During Exposure to Natural and Urban Environments 11: 201-230. J Environ Psychol. 1991;11:201–30.

31.   Babisch W. Transportation noise and cardiovascular risk: Updated Review and synthesis of epidemiological studies indicate that the evidence has increased. Noise Health. 2006;8(30):1–29.

32.   Barceló MA, Varga D, Tobias A, Diaz J, Linares C, Saez M. Long term effects of traffic noise on mortality in the city of Barcelona, 2004–2007. Environ Res. 2016 May;147:193–206.

33.   Tobías A, Recio A, Díaz J, Linares C. Noise levels and cardiovascular mortality: a case-crossover analysis. Eur J Prev Cardiol. 2015;22(4):496–502.

34.   Tobías A, Díaz J, Recio A, Linares C. Traffic noise and risk of mortality from diabetes. Acta Diabetol. 2015;52(1):187–8.

35.   Tobías A, Recio A, Díaz J, Linares C. Does traffic noise influence respiratory mortality? Eur Respir J. 2014;44(3):797–9.

36.   Tobías A, Recio A, Díaz J, Linares C. Health impact assessment of traffic noise in Madrid (Spain). Environ Res. 2015;137:136–40.

37.   Hänninen O, Knol AB, Jantunen M, Lim T-A, Conrad A, Rappolder M, et al. Environmental Burden of Disease in Europe: Assessing Nine Risk Factors in Six Countries. Environ Health Perspect. 2014;122(5):439–46.

38.   García Sanz B, Garrido FJ. La contaminación acústica en nuestras ciudades [Internet]. Barcelona: Fundación 'La

Caixa'; 2003 [cited 2015 Oct 8]. 254 p. (Colección Estudios Sociales). Available from: https://obrasocial.lacaixa.es/deployedfiles/obrasocial/Est aticos/pdf/Estudios_sociales/es12_esp.pdf

39. Weichbold V, Holzer A, Newesely G, Stephan K. Results from high-frequency hearing screening in 14- to 15-year old adolescents and their relation to self-reported exposure to loud music. Int J Audiol. 2012;51(9):650–4.

40. Wilsont WJ, Herbstein N. The role of music intensity in aerobics: implications for hearing conservation. J Am Acad Audiol. 2003;14(1):29–38.

41. Henderson D, Bielefeld EC, Harris KC, Hu BH. The role of oxidative stress in noise-induced hearing loss. Ear Hear. 2006;27(1):1–19.

42. Ohlemiller KK. Recent findings and emerging questions in cochlear noise injury. Hear Res. 2008;245(1–2):5–17.

43. Borg E, Canlon B, Engström B. Noise-induced hearing loss. Literature review and experiments in rabbits. Morphological and electrophysiological features, exposure parameters and temporal factors, variability and interactions. Scand Audiol Suppl. 1995;40:1–147.

44. Roberts LE, Eggermont JJ, Caspary DM, Shore SE, Melcher JR, Kaltenbach JA. Ringing ears: the neuroscience of tinnitus. J Neurosci Off J Soc Neurosci. 2010;30(45):14972–9.

45. Houtgast T, Festen JM. On the auditory and cognitive functions that may explain an individual's elevation of the speech reception threshold in noise. Int J Audiol. 2008;47(6):287–95.

46. Moore BC. Perceptual consequences of cochlear hearing loss and their implications for the design of hearing aids. Ear Hear. 1996 Apr;17(2):133–61.

47. Pienkowski M, Eggermont JJ. Reversible long-term changes in auditory processing in mature auditory cortex in the

absence of hearing loss induced by passive, moderate-level sound exposure. Ear Hear. 2012;33(3):305–14.

48. Baron NS, Segerstad YH af. Cross-cultural patterns in mobile-phone use: public space and reachability in Sweden, the USA and Japan. New Media Soc. 2010;12(1):13–34.

49. Hygge S, Evans GW, Bullinger M. A prospective study of some effects of aircraft noise on cognitive performance in schoolchildren. Psychol Sci. 2002;13(5):469–74.

50. Stansfeld SA, Berglund B, Clark C, Lopez-Barrio I, Fischer P, Ohrström E, et al. Aircraft and road traffic noise and children's cognition and health: a cross-national study. Lancet Lond Engl. 2005;365(9475):1942–9.

51. AC 91-36D - Visual Flight Rules (VFR) Flight Near Noise-Sensitive Areas – Document Information [Internet]. [cited 2016 Jul 12]. Available from: https://www.faa.gov/regulations_policies/advisory_circul ars/index.cfm/go/document.information/documentID/23 156

52. Dutilleux G. Anthropogenic outdoor sound and wildlife: it's not just bioacoustics! Société Fr Acoust Acustics 2012 Apr 2012 Nantes Fr [Internet]. 2012 [cited 2015 Jul 28]; Available from: https://hal.archives-ouvertes.fr/hal-00810795/

53. Figueroa Hernández DD, González Sánchez DF. Relación entre la pérdida de la audición y la exposición al ruido recreativo. Biomics®. 2011;15–21.

54. Niemann H, Maschke C. WHO LARES. Final report. Noise effects and morbidity [Internet]. World Health Organization; 2004 [cited 2015 May 6]. Available from: http://en.wikipedia.org/w/index.php?title=Health_effects _from_noise&oldid=656285611

55. Recomendaciones de buenas prácticas acústicas. Día Internacional de Concienciación sobre el Ruido. Rev Acústica. 2005;36(1):46.

56. Izadi F, Mohseni R, Daneshi A, Sandughdar N. Determination of Fundamental Frequency and Voice Intensity in Iranian Men and Women Aged Between 18 and 45 Years. J Voice. 2012;26(3):336–40.

57. Aronson A. Clinical Voice Disorders. New York, NY: Thieme; 1990.

58. Elliot C, Adams RJ, Sockalingam S. Communication Patterns and Assumptions of Differing Cultural Groups in the United States [Internet]. 1999 [cited 2016 Aug 23]. Available from: http://www.awesomelibrary.org/mul ticulturaltoolkit-patterns.html

59. Kaplan RB. Cultural Thought Patterns in Inter-Cultural Education. Lang Learn. 1966;16 (1-2):11–25.

60. Velo V. Cross-Cultural Management. Business Expert Press; 2011. 231 p.

61. Karpf A. The Human Voice: The Story of a Remarkable Talent. Bloomsbury Publishing; 2011.

62. Bastian RW, Thomas JP. Do Talkativeness and Vocal Loudness Correlate With Laryngeal Pathology? A Study of the Vocal Overdoer/Underdoer Continuum. J Voice [Internet]. 2015 [cited 2016 Jul 8]; Available from: http://linkinghub.elsevier.com/retrieve/pii/S08921997150 01447

63. Yano J, Ichimura K, Hoshino T, Nozue M. Personality factors in pathogenesis of polyps and nodules of vocal cords. Auris Nasus Larynx. 1982;9(2):105–10.

64. Roy N, Holt KI, Redmond S, Muntz H. Behavioral Characteristics of Children With Vocal Fold Nodules. J Voice. 2007;21(2):157–68.

65. Yamada H. Different Games, Different Rules: Why Americans and Japanese Misunderstand Each Other (New York: Oxford University Press, 1997).

66. De Monserrat i Nonó, J, Orri Plaja, A, Corselles Corbella, C, Mer Santamaría, M. El uso profesional de la voz [Internet]. Departamento de Empresa y Empleo. 2012 [cited 2016 Jan

21]. 20 p. Available from: http://www.activamutua.es/wp-content/uploads/2015/06/US_PROFESSIONAL_VEU_cast.pdf

67.   Universidad del País Vasco. La voz humana [Internet]. [cited 2016 Jan 21]. Available from: http://www.ehu.eus/acustica/espanol/musica/vohues/vohues.html

68.   ISO 9921. Ergonomics – assessment of speech communication. Geneva; 2003 [Internet]. [cited 2015 May 5]. Available from: https://www.iso.org/obp/ui/#iso:std:33589:en

69.   Mallory EB, Miller VR. A Possible Basis for the Association of Voice Characteristics and Personality Traits. Speech Monogr. 1958 Nov;25(4):255.

70.   Eisler RM, Miller PM, Hersen M. Components of assertive behavior. J Clin Psychol. 1973;29(3):295–9.

71.   Rose YJ, Tryon WW. Judgments of Assertive Behavior as a Function of Speech Loudness, Latency, Content, Gestures, Inflection, and Sex. Behav Modif. 1979;3(1):112–23.

72.   Educar sin gritar. Guillermo Ballenato Prieto. Ed. La esfera de los libros. 2007.

73.   Amazi DK, Garber SR. The Lombard sign as a function of age and task. J Speech Hear Res. 1982;25(4):581–5.

74.   Mireia Canals, Mar Cerdà. El cuento de hablar sin gritar. Primera edición. Barcelona, España: Miguel A. Salvatella, S.A.; 2009.

75.   Truby HM. Prenatal sound transmission and exceptional antennae [Internet]. [cited 2015 Apr 24]. Available from: http://scitation.aip.org/content/asa/journal/jasa/62/S1/10.1121/1.2016439

76.   Roy N, Merrill RM, Thibeault S, Parsa RA, Gray SD, Smith EM. Prevalence of voice disorders in teachers and the general population. J Speech Lang Hear Res JSLHR. 2004;47(2):281–93.

77. Pearsons K, Bennett K, Fidell S. Speech levels in various noise environments. U.S. Environmental Protection Agency Report EPA-600/1-77-025, 1977. Available through the National Technical Information Service, Springfield, Virginia.y [Internet]. 1977 [cited 2015 May 5]. Available from: http://nepis.epa.gov

78. Södersten M, Granqvist S, Hammarberg B, Szabo A. Vocal behavior and vocal loading factors for preschool teachers at work studied with binaural DAT recordings. J Voice Off J Voice Found. 2002;16(3):356–71.

79. Williams NR. Occupational groups at risk of voice disorders: a review of the literature. Occup Med. 2003;53(7):456–60.

80. Pérez Fernández, CA, Preciado López, J. Nódulos de las cuerdas vocales. Factores de riesgo en los docentes. Estudio de casos y controles. Acta Otorrinolaringológica Esp. 2003;54:253–60.

81. Hick CB, Tharpe AM. Listening effort and fatigue in school-age children with and without hearing loss. J Speech Lang Hear Res JSLHR. 2002;45(3):573–84.

82. Anderson Gosselin P, Gagne´ J-P. Older Adults Expend More Listening Effort Than Young Adults Recognizing Speech in Noise. J Speech Lang Hear Res. 2011;54(3):944.

83. Speech understanding and aging. Working Group on Speech Understanding and Aging. Committee on Hearing, Bioacoustics, and Biomechanics, Commission on Behavioral and Social Sciences and Education, National Research Council. J Acoust Soc Am. 1988;83(3):859–95.

84. Nabelek AK, Tucker FM, Letowski TR. Toleration of background noises: relationship with patterns of hearing aid use by elderly persons. J Speech Hear Res. 1991;34(3):679–85.

85. Recker KL, Edwards BW. The Effect of Presentation Level on Normal-Hearing and Hearing-Impaired Listeners' Acceptable Speech and Noise Levels. J Am Acad Audiol. 2013;24(1):17-25 9p.

86.   Hodgetts WE, Rieger JM, Szarko RA. The effects of listening environment and earphone style on preferred listening levels of normal hearing adults using an MP3 player. Ear Hear. 2007;28(3):290–7.

87.   Mackersie CL, Cones H. Subjective and psychophysiological indices of listening effort in a competing-talker task. J Am Acad Audiol. 2011 Feb;22(2):113–22.

88.   Gates GA, Mills JH. Presbycusis. Lancet Lond Engl. 2005;366(9491):1111–20.

89.   van Rooij JC, Plomp R. Auditive and cognitive factors in speech perception by elderly listeners. III. Additional data and final discussion. J Acoust Soc Am. 1992;91(2):1028–33.

90.   Helfer KS, Vargo M. Speech recognition and temporal processing in middle-aged women. J Am Acad Audiol. 2009;20(4):264–71.

91.   Morrell CH, Gordon-Salant S, Pearson JD, Brant LJ, Fozard JL. Age- and gender-specific reference ranges for hearing level and longitudinal changes in hearing level. J Acoust Soc Am. 1996;100(4 Pt 1):1949–67.

92.   Degeest S, Keppler H, Corthals P. The Effect of Age on Listening Effort. J Speech Lang Hear Res. 2015;58(5):1592.

93.   Veneman CE, Gordon-Salant S, Matthews LJ, Dubno JR. Age and Measurement Time-of-Day Effects on Speech Recognition in Noise: Ear Hear. 2013;34(3):288–99.

94.   Gilles A, Ihtijarevic B, Wouters K, Van de Heyning P. Using prophylactic antioxidants to prevent noise-induced hearing damage in young adults: a protocol for a double-blind, randomized controlled trial. Trials. 2014;15:110.

95.   Al calor del amor en un bar. Gabinete Caligari. 1986. Sello: DRO-Tres cipreses.

96.   Tóth MA, Lecumberri MLG, Tang Y, Cooke M. A corpus of noise-induced word misperceptions for Spanish. J Acoust Soc Am. 2015;137(2):EL184–EL189.

97.   Culling JF. Energetic and Informational Masking in a Simulated Restaurant Environment. In: Moore BCJ,

Patterson RD, Winter IM, Carlyon RP, Gockel HE, editors. Basic Aspects of Hearing [Internet]. New York, NY: Springer New York; 2013 [cited 2015 Apr 24]. p. 511–8. Available from: http://link.springer.com/10.1007/978-1-4614-1590-9_56

98. Navarro MPN, Pimentel RL. Speech interference in food courts of shopping centres. Appl Acoust. 2007;68(3):364–75.

99. Lazarus H. Prediction of verbal communication in noise—A development of generalized SIL curves and the quality of communication (Part 2). Appl Acoust. 1987;20(4):245–61.

100. Brumm H, Zollinger A. The evolution of the Lombard effect: 100 years of psychoacoustic research. Behaviour. 2011;148(11–13):1173–98.

101. Rindel JH. Acoustical capacity as a means of noise control in eating establishments. Proc BNAM [Internet]. 2012 [cited 2015 Apr 28]; Available from: http://www.researchgate.net/profile/Jens_Rindel/publica tion/265888641_Acoustical_capacity_as_a_means_of_noi se_control_in_eating_establishments/links/54201ddd0cf2 218008d44116.pdf

102. Vera Gurarinos G, Yebra Calleja M, Calzado Estepa E. Condiciones acústicas en bares-restaurantes: una primera aproximación al establecimiento de la 'distancia mínima de confort' entre mesas. 46° Congr Esp Acústica Encuentro Ibérico Acústica Eur Symp Virtual Acoust Ambisonics Valencia Spain. 2015;

103. Strait DL, Kraus N. Can You Hear Me Now? Musical Training Shapes Functional Brain Networks for Selective Auditory Attention and Hearing Speech in Noise. Front Psychol [Internet]. 2011 [cited 2016 Jan 22];2(113). Available from: http://journal.frontiersin.org/article/10.3389/fpsyg.2011. 00113/abstract

104. Zhang C, Arnott SR, Rabaglia C, Avivi-Reich M, Qi J, Wu X, et al. Attentional modulation of informational masking on

early cortical representations of speech signals. Hear Res. 2016;331:119–30.

105. Zhang C, Lu L, Wu X, Li L. Attentional modulation of the early cortical representation of speech signals in informational or energetic masking. Brain Lang. 2014;135:85–95.

106. Cherry EC. Some Experiments on the Recognition of Speech, with One and with Two Ears. J Acoust Soc Am. 1953;25(5):975–9.

107. Plude DJ, Enns JT, Brodeur D. The development of selective attention: a life-span overview. Acta Psychol (Amst). 1994;86(2–3):227–72.

108. Desjardins JL, Doherty KA. Age-related changes in listening effort for various types of masker noises. Ear Hear. 2013;34(3):261–72.

109. Shield BM, Dockrell JE. The effects of noise on children at school: a review. Build Acoust. 2003;10(2):97–116.

110. Preciado-López J, Pérez-Fernández C, Calzada-Uriondo M, Preciado-Ruiz P. Epidemiological Study of Voice Disorders Among Teaching Professionals of La Rioja, Spain. J Voice. 2008;22(4):489–508.

111. de Medeiros AM, Assunção AÁ, Barreto SM. Absenteeism due to voice disorders in female teachers: a public health problem. Int Arch Occup Environ Health. 2012;85(8):853–64.

112. Kaarlela-Tuomaala A, Helenius R, Keskinen E, Hongisto V. Effects of acoustic environment on work in private office rooms and open-plan offices - longitudinal study during relocation. Ergonomics. 2009;52(11):1423–44.

113. Pierrette M, Parizet E, Chevret P, Chatillon J. Noise effect on comfort in open-space offices: development of an assessment questionnaire. Ergonomics. 2015;58(1):96–106.

114. Schlittmeier SJ, Liebl A. The effects of intelligible irrelevant background speech in offices - cognitive disturbance, annoyance, and solutions. Facilities. 2015;33(1/2):75–61.

115. ISO 3382-3:2012. Acoustics – measurement of room acoustic parameters – Part 3: open-plan offices. Geneva, Switzerland: International Organization for Standardization; 2012.

116. Huang R-H, Shih Y-N. Effects of background music on concentration of workers. Work. 2011;38(4):383-387 5p.

117. Shih Y-N, Huang R-H, Chiang H-Y. Background music: Effects on attention performance. Work. 2012;42(4):573-578 6p.

118. Rusnock CF, Bush PM. An evaluation of restaurant noise levels and contributing factors. J Occup Environ Hyg. 2012;9(6):D108-113.

119. Lebo CP, Smith MF, Mosher ER, Jelonek SJ, Schwind DR, Decker KE, et al. Restaurant noise, hearing loss, and hearing aids. West J Med. 1994 Jul;161(1):45–9.

120. To W, Chung A. Noise in restaurants: Levels and mathematical model. Noise Health. 2014;16(73):368–73.

121. Nelson JP. Highway noise and property values: A survey of recent evidence. J Transp Econ Pol. 1982;16:117–38.

122. Roy N, Merrill RM, Gray SD, Smith EM. Voice disorders in the general population: prevalence, risk factors, and occupational impact. The Laryngoscope. 2005;115(11):1988–95.

123. Smith E, Verdolini K, Gray S, Nichols S, Lemke J, Barkmeier J, et al. Effect of voice disorders on quality of life. J Med Speech-Lang Pathol. 1996;4(4):223–44.

124. Cohen SM, Kim J, Roy N, Asche C, Courey M. Direct health care costs of laryngeal diseases and disorders. The Laryngoscope. 2012;122(7):1582–8.

125. Shield B. Evaluation of the social and economic costs of hearing impairment. Hear-It AISBL. 2006;1–202.

DEFINITIONS, ABBREVIATIONS AND ACRONYMS

- ANL: acceptable noise level.

- dB: decibel. Unit of acoustic intensity, equivalent to one tenth of a bel.

- dB(A): decibel on the A-weighted scale (scale closest to the human ear).

- Hyperacusis: reduction of tolerable noise levels for the ears.

- Hz: Hertz. Unit of frequency or tone of the sound.

- OECD: Organization for Economic Co-operation and Development.

- RT: reverberation time.

- Tinnitus: buzzing or beeps that are heard in the ears, but do not come from an external sound source.

- WHO: World Health Organisation.